I0455738

Getting Started with Breastfeeding

For Catholic Mothers

By Gina Peterson

Copyright © 2014 Gina Peterson

All rights reserved.

ISBN-10: 1493796372
ISBN-13: 978-1493796373

Table of Contents

Acknowledgements

Thank you, Dominic, for your love and support and for taking the beautiful pictures of Leia for the front and back cover. Thank you, Lukas, Ethan, Benjamin, Samuel, and Leia for our wonderful breastfeeding relationships over the years. Thank you, Pam, for founding the Catholic Nursing Mothers League, for including me in its inception, and for passing the leadership of it over to me five years ago. Thank you, Sheila, for all the work you have done to spread the good news of ecological breastfeeding, for your mentorship, and for your help with proofreading my book. Thank you, Grace, Tiz, and Andrea for being part of the Catholic Nursing Mothers League Board of Directors and for your many insights and contributions to CNML. Thank you, Maureen, Marian, Judith, Pam, and Andrea for sharing your personal breastfeeding stories. Thank you, Kelley, Pam, Andrea and John for your help with proofreading. Thank you, members of the Catholic Nursing Mothers League Yahoo group, Facebook page and readers and contributors of the blog, for being part of this ministry.

Foreword

by Pamela H. Pilch

Fifty years ago, when the now well-known mother-to-mother-support organization La Leche League (LLL) was started, breastfeeding was not only out of fashion – it was nearly extinct! At that time, more than 80% of mothers bottle-fed their newborns using formula (so-called because it had to be mixed from a special recipe, which was considered more scientific than nursing). Those who desired to breastfeed received little encouragement or support from their doctors, families or friends. Hospital practices were so burdensome that even those determined few often found it difficult to nurse past the first few weeks.

Times have certainly changed. A recent study revealed that 72% of mothers in the U.S. breastfeed their babies at least briefly.[1] Birthing and postpartum practices such as rooming-in with newborns and delayed introduction of bottles and pacifiers have become more common. Mothers have a choice of breastfeeding support services, including professional lactation consultants, LLL groups, hospital-based mothers' meetings and WIC peer counselors. Articles (of varying quality) on breastfeeding periodically turn up in newspapers and parenting magazines. Even the U.S. government has gotten into the act, having produced a controversial but widely-publicized campaign proclaiming that "Babies are born to be breastfed!"[2] A few mothers who are ambivalent about breastfeeding report feeling pressured by the many voices encouraging nursing as the healthiest option for their babies.

And yet...even with all this publicity and support, breastfeeding rates for babies at 6 months of age lag discouragingly behind the U.S. government's public health goals. Even fewer are nursing at the age of one year, the minimum length of time recommended by the American Academy of Pediatrics for optimal infant health. Mothers who nurse their children for two years and beyond, in accordance with World Health Organization guidelines, hardly make it onto the general public's radar, though a determined sub-culture of "extended breastfeeding" mothers exists, if one knows where to look. Most Americans only encounter toddler nursing through sensational, and (usually) inaccurate, portrayals in movies, TV dramas or daytime talk shows.

Why, then, with so much medical, scientific and government support, do not more mothers choose to nurse, or choose to nurse longer?

In their book *Breastfeeding Made Simple: Seven Natural Laws for Nursing Mothers*, Nancy Mohrbacher, IBCLC, and Kathleen Kendall-Tackett, Ph.D., IBCLC,[3] explore modern cultural barriers to breastfeeding. They describe how the rise of bottle-feeding in generations past has led to general ignorance about the way natural breastfeeding actually works. In the 1940s, 50s and 60s, a cultural preference for "scientific" mothering (replacing natural processes with new, "improved" man-made technology) led many to apply bottle-feeding management techniques, such as scheduled every-four-hour feedings, to breastfeeding. Continued adherence to these principles contributes to breastfeeding failure for many moms even today. In addition, the authors explore the pervasive commercial pressures that undermine breastfeeding, such as unethical formula marketing, and the continuing lack of education among health care professionals on the needs of breastfeeding couples.

Additionally, they outline a number of beliefs about babies, parenting, and sexuality, common among some Christian parents, including many Catholics, which negatively affect breastfeeding initiation and duration. Examples include the belief that strict feeding schedules help prevent "spoiling", that babies cry in order to manipulate their parents and that proper discipline begins early with "showing the baby who's boss". Some parenting organizations (including some Christian groups) advocate letting the baby "cry it out" between scheduled feedings and before going to sleep, practices which are, in fact, detrimental to the nursing relationship. Certain beliefs about modesty and the proper use of the body, appropriate in many other contexts, may also be a stumbling block for nursing moms, who may feel that breastfeeding is too limiting, requires them to stay at home too much, or prevents them from participating meaningfully in church or social functions. This is especially true if their own priest or fellow parishioners frown on nursing children at Mass or other parish gatherings.

Finally, some Christian childcare experts inadvertently undermine breastfeeding by emphasizing the primacy of the marital relationship to such an extent that the mother's efforts to meet her child's legitimate needs through breastfeeding on cue (also called "responsive breastfeeding"), or co-sleeping, are seen as damaging to the Christian marriage.

Although Catholic mothers have a great deal of Church support for their role and vocation in general, they are subject to the same cultural pressures experienced by all U.S. mothers in regard to breastfeeding. In addition, they often find themselves directed by friends, family or the media to certain rigid "Christian" parenting resources of the type described above, due to a perceived lack of resources reflecting a distinctly Catholic perspective on breastfeeding and the parenting of young children. [4]

Catholic mothers who faithfully follow Church teaching by avoiding the use of artificial contraception sometimes face even more challenges when their use of natural family planning (NFP) is complicated by postpartum irregularity in their fertility cycles. Breastfeeding mothers who use NFP often report an inclination to wean their babies early just to facilitate a return to more familiar NFP rules after regular cycles return. These mothers need special information, encouragement and support by knowledgeable teachers, as well as from other similarly-situated moms.

Catholic teaching and tradition offer lots of support for mothers who want to breastfeed their babies, and Catholic resources are available. Still, many Catholic moms don't always know where to turn for faithful and reliable advice. Catholic moms need Catholic support! And Catholic support could be the key to helping more moms and babies enjoy the terrific benefits nursing can bring.

In a presentation to health care professionals in Detroit, Michigan (spring 2006), IBCLC Diane Wiessinger[5] encouraged the creation of breastfeeding "mini-cultures" as an effective way to increase breastfeeding rates among various groups of women. A "mini-culture" is a group of mothers who share something important in common. It could be their religion, their neighborhood, their school or professional affiliation – anything that makes the women in the group feel that they share a common bond. When women gather in groups with other like-minded mothers who breastfeed, it increases their confidence in their choice to nurse their own babies. Feeling they are not alone in their decision to breastfeed helps them persevere through challenges and difficulties.

Practically speaking, where can a Catholic mom turn for support?

This book, written by co-Founder and Executive Director of the Catholic Nursing Mothers League and IBCLC, Gina Peterson, is the answer to this question!

Getting Started with Breastfeeding: For Catholic Mothers combines the basic practical information new mothers need to get breastfeeding off to a good start and deal with common challenges, with a wealth of beautiful spiritual resources and encouragement for nursing mothers at every stage.

In this book, Gina recognizes that breastfeeding is both a physical and a profoundly spiritual activity. She has offered her considerable expertise in professional lactation consulting to the benefit of her readers. But she has also shared openly her personal experiences as a breastfeeding mother, and especially as a devout and serious practicing Catholic. She sensitively portrays the joys and challenges Catholic moms encounter and offers a wealth of suggestions for every problem - practical, emotional or spiritual.

I especially appreciate this book's unabashed support for the practice of full ecological breastfeeding, as advocated for the past 30 years by breastfeeding advocate and NFP pioneers Sheila and John Kippley.

And I know that this book will help many mothers discover the blessing of involvement in the Catholic Nursing Mothers League, an organization dedicated to building up the "mini-culture of breastfeeding" that is proper to the Catholic Church.

With more education and encouragement, the entire Catholic community can help increase breastfeeding rates among Catholic moms. This will bring real benefits, physical, mental, emotional, and even spiritual, to our children, mothers, families, communities and society itself. Breastfeeding really does make a difference, and as Catholics, we have a great tradition of support for the family to guide us in our efforts. I know this book will make a huge contribution to this tradition.

[1]U.S. Department of Health and Human Services, Centers for Disease Control, 2005 National Immunization Survey: Breastfeeding Practices:

[2]http://www.4woman.gov/breastfeeding/index.cfm?page =Campaign

[3]http://www.breastfeedingmadesimple.com.

[4]Dr. Gregory Popcak, Catholic author and psychotherapist, has written a very informative paper outlining the various trends in Christian parenting advice and has detailed their theological origin. He proposes a distinctly Catholic approach to parenting. A copy of this paper can be obtained by contacting Dr. Popcak. Popcak's general theory about a theologically-consistent "Catholic" approach to childrearing is also found in his book, Parenting with Grace: The Catholic Parents Guide to Raising (Almost) Perfect Kids, available at http://www.exceptionalmarriages.com.

[5]http://www.wiessinger.baka.com/bfing/index.html

A Nursing Mother's Prayer

Thank you, God, for this baby, your gift of life, marriage, and especially for your wonderful gift of breastfeeding. Sometimes I feel tired and overwhelmed by the demands of motherhood; sometimes I feel like I am constantly nursing day and night, that I have not time to get anything else done and that others who need me don't get what they need because of the demands of this season of my life. Help me to remember that I am following Your special plan for mothers and babies, and that You will give me the grace to do all that you want me to do and to share Your love with my family. Help me to feel Your presence as I try my best to cooperate with Your plan. Amen.

Saint Pope John Paul II on Breastfeeding

May 12, 1995

"...[Breastfeeding] benefits the child and helps to create the closeness and maternal bonding so necessary for healthy child development. So human and natural is this bond that the Psalms use the image of the infant at its mother's breast as a picture of God's care for man..."

Introduction

Congratulations on the birth of your baby! As you embark (or continue) on the exciting journey of breastfeeding and motherhood, I hope you will find this book a useful and encouraging companion. This book is unique in that it was written specifically with the Catholic mother in mind, considering her unique needs and desires. It wholeheartedly embraces all aspects of Catholic Church teaching, aims to help mothers incorporate Catholic spirituality and practice into all they do, and introduces the Catholic Nursing Mothers League, an organization especially for the support of Catholic moms. This book also wholeheartedly embraces the practice of ecological breastfeeding, God's special plan for mothering and child spacing. This book was written by a Catholic nursing mother, even while nursing a baby in arms!

Here mothers will learn the basics of breastfeeding and solutions to a few of the more common breastfeeding problems and receive encouragement for living the ecological breastfeeding lifestyle. Mothers who have a nursing mothers group in their parish will find this book a useful resource for their group.

This book is NOT intended as a medical resource or as a comprehensive reference text on all aspects of breastfeeding. If you need more information or have a specific breastfeeding concern, please seek the advice of a trained breastfeeding counselor or international board certified lactation consultant (IBCLC). This book is not intended for diagnosis or treatment of medical conditions. Please see your health care provider for medical advice.

One of the most difficult challenges of writing a breastfeeding or mothering book is the acknowledgment that many mothers give birth, and attempt to breastfeed under less-than-ideal circumstances. In our society today it is difficult or even impossible for some mothers to nurse. When breastfeeding does not go well, you may feel sad, disappointed, depressed, or even angry, and experience shame or guilt. This book is in no way intended to increase your pain if you are in this situation. You may have made heroic efforts to be available to your baby, to provide your milk for him, and to build a satisfying breastfeeding relationship in spite of significant limitations. In our mothering journey, we must all realize that we do the best we can with the resources, knowledge and support that we have at any given time. One of the central tenets of the Catholic Nursing Mothers League is that a mother's presence to her baby is the most important thing, and that whether or not she breastfeeds, or breastfeeds fully, or practices ecological breastfeeding, she is the most precious gift of God to her baby and her family. By trying to build up communities of support for mothers, and especially for those trying to breastfeed and mother within the Catholic community, we hope to ease the path of all mothers and to strengthen the family in every good way.

Chapter 1: Breastfeeding Basics

Benefits of Breastfeeding

In our world today, society SEEMS to emphasize the importance of children and the importance of motherhood, but the emphasis in the mainstream society is on the materialistic aspects of these things - having the right THINGS, the right daycare, the right equipment, etc. However in the Church, we recognize the importance of the human person, and also the way in which God's creation, when understood rightly, supports the optimal development - physical, mental, psychological, emotional and spiritual - of each person.

Research not only shows that breastfeeding has many benefits to babies, but also that there are risks to not breastfeeding. Non-breastfed babies are at increased risk of developing the following: dental and vision problems, allergies, Crohn's disease, leukemia, type 1 and type 2 diabetes, ear infections, severe diarrhea, obesity, ulcerative colitis, SIDS (Sudden Infant Death Syndrome), osteoporosis, necrotizing enterocolitis, lower IQ, and heart disease (*The Baby Book, Revised and Updated Edition 2013*, p.135). Breastfeeding has a profound effect on your baby's health!

Breast milk is a living fluid, so it changes its chemical proportions in response to different circumstances. If your baby is born prematurely, the proportions of protein and fat will change to accommodate a not-yet-full-term baby. Also, if you develop an illness, your body makes antibodies against that particular virus or bacteria, and those wonderful antibodies are then transferred to the baby via breast milk to protect your little one. When a toddler is still nursing but nursing less often than a younger baby, your milk compensates by increasing its concentration of immunities to continue protecting your toddler. In addition, the type of fats in your diet influences the types of fats present in your milk, so increasing your omega-3 fatty acid consumption is good for both of you. Breast milk is a great way for your baby to experience the different flavors of foods you eat. Breast milk is more than "just" milk!

Breastfeeding has many benefits for babies, but there are also great benefits for mothers as well. God's plan always works for the good of all involved in a relationship. So when He designed breastfeeding to benefit babies, of course, He didn't leave mothers out! Breastfeeding reduces your risk of ovarian cancer, breast cancer, cervical cancer, rheumatoid arthritis, and metabolic syndrome. If you have insulin dependent diabetes, you may find you will need less insulin while breastfeeding. Breastfeeding helps protect against high blood pressure, osteoporosis, and fractures, too (*The Baby Book, Revised and Updated Edition 2013*, p. 135). One of the focuses of this book, ecological breastfeeding, can extend your amenorrhea (no periods) and postpartum infertility naturally for months - and sometimes years - which can give you and baby more time to bond and give you more time to adjust to your new addition.

In addition, breastfeeding helps your uterus return to its original size sooner and with less risk of postpartum hemorrhage. Because you burn approximately 500 more calories per day when nursing than when not pregnant or nursing, you are more likely to return to your pre-pregnancy weight. The hormones produced during breastfeeding - prolactin and oxytocin - not only help your body make milk but also help you relax. The time you spend nursing your baby helps you bond and feel close to your baby. Breastfeeding is good for you both physically and emotionally.

Breastfeeding is also great for your pocketbook, for the environment and for the sanity of the mother since there is no need to prepare formula or wash bottles. Breast milk is free. Because many women experience amenorrhea for several months or years while breastfeeding, there is less waste from feminine hygiene products. The diapers of exclusively breastfed babies smell more pleasant than diapers of babies not breastfeeding (good for your home environment!). Breastfeeding makes night time parenting easier and traveling easier on mom, dad and baby because breast milk is readily available.

As Catholics, we believe that there is more to life than just our physical existence. Just as breastfeeding has many great physical benefits for the baby and mother, it also provides wonderful spiritual benefits as well. Mothering your baby at the breast helps your baby experience the unconditional love of Jesus in a very tangible way. You are your baby's first glimpse of God. When you nurse him in the middle of the night, you are showing your baby that God will always take care of him. When you respond to his cries and put him to your breast, you are not only nourishing him physically but sharing God's comfort.

There are spiritual benefits for you, too. God gives you special graces through the sacrament of Holy Matrimony and through your vocation of motherhood (whether it be by birth or adoption) to follow God's will for you in this time of your life. Just as on some days you might not get a long shower or enough sleep, on other days God will want you to put up your feet, sip a glass of cold water, and enjoy some quiet time in His presence while nursing your sweet baby!

Preparing to Breastfeed

Mothers today are faced with so many sources of information: doctors' advice, books, magazines, websites, Facebook pages, the experiences of friends and relatives! One of the first steps in preparing to breastfeed is to read about breastfeeding from reliable sources. Two excellent internet sites are www.catholicbreastfeeding.org and www.askdrears.com. The former offers an online support community via Yahoo groups and Facebook which can be invaluable if you live in a rural area or just do not know many nursing mothers. *The Baby Book, Revised and Updated Edition: Everything You Need to Know About Your Baby from Birth to Age Two (2013)* by Dr. William Sears, Martha Sears, Dr. Robert Sears, and Dr. James Sears is a very good, comprehensive book about breastfeeding, baby care, and attachment parenting. The authors are Catholic and even discuss the benefits of breastfeeding for spacing babies!

Besides reading quality Internet sites and books, locating a good breastfeeding support network before your baby is born is another important step. Even though you can read a lot about breastfeeding, you really cannot learn it solely through reading a book. Speaking to mothers in person about their real life experiences is an excellent way to learn.

There are different options depending on what type of support you are seeking. If someone has started a nursing mothers group in your parish, you can fellowship, pray and discuss breastfeeding, natural family planning, Catholic motherhood, and gentle parenting with other like-minded

Catholic women at their functions. If there isn't currently a group at your church, consider starting one yourself. There are resources on the CNML website that will assist you.

If you are looking for more specific information on breastfeeding management, you can attend breastfeeding support meetings in your community during and after pregnancy. They are usually led by a trained breastfeeding counselor or lactation consultant.

If you find yourself facing complex breastfeeding issues, International Board Certified Lactation Consultants (IBCLCs) can work one on one with you to troubleshoot the problems and to help you achieve your breastfeeding goals. IBCLCs, as other health care professionals, normally charge for their services. However, most mothers will tell you that the fee is well worth it! Also, don't forget about finding a breastfeeding friendly health care provider with whom you feel comfortable. Ask friends and family for recommendations and consider interviewing your top choices.

Last but not least, husbands are some of the best supporters of breastfeeding, so keep him involved in all the reading and classes you take.

In terms of practicalities, many nursing moms find nursing bras indispensable. You'll want to pick a bra that is comfortable, not too tight and big enough to allow for an increase in breast size when your milk comes in. Breast size can increase even one whole cup size after the baby is born and your milk comes in! Sometimes underwire bras can contribute to plugged ducts so picking a bra without underwire would be best if possible. Many maternity stores have staff that can assist you in finding the best fitting bra.

Breasts and nipples of all sizes are perfectly suited to breastfeed successfully! However, some types, such as inverted nipples, can make breastfeeding a little more challenging in the beginning. If you think you have inverted nipples, you may consider asking your health care provider to confirm. If you have inverted nipples, you can still nurse your baby! You may just need a little extra help with latch after your baby is born. Some women have found success using a nipple everter during pregnancy or after their baby is born to drawn an inverted nipple out.

There is no need to do anything to prepare your breasts for breastfeeding. The good news is that pregnancy itself prepares a woman's body perfectly well for breastfeeding. You can be confident that just as your body knows how to grow your baby perfectly according to God's plan, your breasts know how to grow and prepare to nurture your baby soon after birth!

Childbirth and Breastfeeding

First of all, no matter what type of birth you end up having - natural, medicated, vaginal, cesarean - you will most likely be able to breastfeed your baby. Even after a difficult or traumatic childbirth, breastfeeding can bring about a wonderful experience of healing and bonding with a newborn, most of the time quickly and effectively. The vast majority - experts say ninety-five percent - of women are physically capable of breastfeeding. That is good news and part of God's design to keep the human race going. That being said, nursing at the breast can be more challenging or delayed in certain circumstances. However, with education and support from other nursing moms, a trained breastfeeding counselor or lactation consultant, breastfeeding will most likely become easier and a natural part of your life as a mother. Breastfeeding is the natural continuation of the cycle that begins with pregnancy and birth.

Two easy ways to increase your chances of having the best birth and early breastfeeding experience as possible are to attend childbirth classes and to read a good childbirth book. Childbirth classes taught independent of hospitals tend to have more information on natural birthing techniques and how to avoid unnecessary interventions. Nursing mother group meetings at your church and breastfeeding support meetings in your community are good places to obtain recommendations for both childbirth books and classes.

Husbands can be great labor coaches. However, many women like having the support of another woman who has given birth herself, such as a friend or mother, in addition to their spouses. There are also labor doulas who have specialized training in supporting and encouraging women in labor. Doulas have been shown in the research evidence to improve mothers' birth experiences and facilitate un-medicated labors and breastfeeding (*The Baby Book, Revised and Updated Edition* 2013, p.22-23). A parish nursing mothers group or a childbirth or breastfeeding class is a good place to ask about local doulas.

It is ideal if the mother can avoid IV fluids during labor and birth. Sometimes too much fluid can cause breast engorgement which makes latching more difficult. Also, certain medications can make babies sleepy at birth. Striving for as un-medicated a birth as possible will help ensure an awake baby, ready to breastfeed.

The first hour after birth is a very special time for bonding and getting baby to the breast before he takes his first long nap. Baths and other post-birth activities can wait until after the first nursing. Hold your baby skin to skin as much as possible in the first hour, and continue lots of loving and holding in the early days postpartum. An un-medicated baby placed on his mother's abdomen soon after birth is actually able to crawl towards the breast and latch on without assistance! There are many unseen hormonal bonding elements going on to help baby get off to a good start with breastfeeding - a beautiful design!

If you do need a cesarean, you can still breastfeed your baby! The key is to try different breastfeeding positions that allow you and your baby to nurse successfully and comfortably while staying away from your incision. Some possibilities: sitting upright with a pillow over your lap to protect your incision, the clutch hold (which is described in more detail in the "Latch and Position" section), and the side-lying position (*The Baby Book, Revised and Updated Edition 2013*, p.191).

Last but not least, writing a birth plan and giving a copy to all birth attendants is another good idea. It is best to let everyone involved in your birth know that you plan to breastfeed and that you do not want your baby to have artificial nipples, bottles, water or formula unless medically necessary. A positive birth experience is always a help to getting breastfeeding off to a good start!

Latch and Positioning

Good latch and positioning help prevent soreness and other breastfeeding issues and also contribute to a good milk supply and encourage adequate drainage of the breasts.

No matter which breastfeeding position you choose, you will want to be tummy to tummy with your baby (if you are using the clutch hold, your baby's tummy should be parallel to your side). Make sure your baby does not need to turn his head to the side to nurse. It is also a good idea not to touch the top of his head while nursing; many babies find this distracting. If your baby's head is slightly tilted back or even if his nose lightly touches your breast, he will be able to breathe; if he can't breathe, he will instinctively stop nursing or you can reposition him (*The Baby Book, Revised and Updated Edition 2013*, p.141).

Wait until he opens his mouth wide and then gently bring him towards you as you latch him onto your breast. He should take in a fair amount of breast tissue, not just your nipple. How much of the areola that is taken in depends upon the size of your areola. If the latch feels uncomfortable or painful, gently insert a clean finger in the corner of his mouth, break the suction, and try latching again. Always break the suction anytime you take baby off the breast to reduce the chance of injury to your nipple. Breastfeeding is supposed to feel pleasant, so cramming your baby on to your breast to latch him isn't the best idea.

To nurse in the side-lying position, lie down on your side and position your baby on his side so the two of you are tummy to tummy and your nipple is level with his nose. You want him to be able to nurse comfortably without his chin being tucked. Propping up a pillow or a rolled up towel behind his back will help stabilize him (*The Baby Book, Revised Edition 2013*, p.142).

If you want to nurse your baby in the cradle hold, hold him horizontally, tummy to tummy with you, with his head in the crook of your arm. The hand of that same arm will help support his back.

The cross cradle hold is similar to the cradle hold, but the opposite hand and arm are used to support the baby's head and back. Instead of baby's head resting in the crook of your arm, it is resting in the palm of your hand (if baby is at left breast, his head is in your right hand). This is a temporary nursing hold that can be used in the early days to allow you more control of your baby's head.

Last but not least, the clutch hold is another nursing position moms enjoy. Hold your baby to the side of your body (his tummy parallel to your side and feet toward the back of the couch or chair). Support his head and neck with the hand nearest to his head on that side of the body and his body between your arm and body. Your breast may be lower than his mouth which can be helpful for large breasted women. This is a good position to use after a cesarean (*The Baby Book, Revised and Updated Edition 2013*, p.142-143).

A picture is worth a thousand words...so if you need more guidance with nursing positions, *The Baby Book, Revised and Updated Edition (2013)* by Dr. William Sears and family has many wonderful pictures. You can also search for pictures of different nursing positions on their website: www.askdrsears.com. An even better idea is to attend your parish's nursing mothers group or a breastfeeding support meeting and observe other mothers breastfeeding their babies. Good latch and positioning help prevent soreness and other breastfeeding issues and also contribute to a good milk supply and encourage adequate drainage of the breasts.

Is Baby Getting Enough?

There are several ways to tell if your baby is getting enough nourishment. As a general guideline, babies need to nurse at least 8-12 times in a 24 hour period. You will know your baby needs to nurse when he sucks his hands, makes mouth movements, roots around as if searching for your breast, or cries. Crying is a late indicator of hunger, so it is best to nurse your baby when he exhibits the earlier signs of hunger. If he is too ravenous or upset, he will have a more difficult time latching. When determining how often to nurse, let your baby lead – not the clock or a schedule. One exception to this would be if your baby is sleepy and not nursing every 2-3 hours during the day and a little less often at night during those first few days. If your baby is sleepy and not nursing often enough, gently try to wake him by undressing him and changing his diaper. Then offer the breast. If his sleepiness continues and he is not nursing at least 8-12 times per 24 hour period, please contact a lactation consultant and your health care provider. Listen to your baby, too, about how long to nurse him. Sometimes he may want to nurse leisurely for long periods of time and others times he will just want a shorter meal. Your baby will let you know what he needs.

When nursing your baby, look for periods of vigorous, slow sucks with periodic pauses. Listen for swallowing and gulping during times of active nursing. Also, look for ear wiggling and jaw movement. These are all signs that your baby is getting your milk and not solely suckling. Follow your baby's lead and let him finish the first breast before you offer him the second side. You can tell that he is finished if he comes off the breast on his own or falls asleep at the breast. Look for satiety - are his hands open and his face serene? Also, by allowing your baby to finish each breast, you help ensure he gets enough of the fatty hind milk that is in greater concentration as the breast gets emptier (*The Baby Book, Revised and Updated Edition 2013*, p.142). Some babies only want to nurse on one side at a particular nursing session or as their regular nursing habit. As you nurse your baby over time, you will discover his own unique nursing style.

After the first three days of life, your baby should have at least 4-6 wet disposable diapers per day or 6-8 wet cloth diapers per day. His stools will change from sticky black to green to brown and then to a yellow mustardy color and seedy texture. You can expect to see at least 2-3 stools (the size of a U.S. quarter or larger) each day after this change is complete. If you notice your baby's stools are regularly green and mucousy, it is possible he might have a foremilk hindmilk imbalance. See the "oversupply" section for ideas on how to balance your milk supply. After six weeks of age, some babies only have a stool once every few days or even once a week; this is normal for healthy, breastfed babies (*The Baby Book, Revised and Updated Edition 2013*, p.150-151).

Do not be alarmed if your baby loses 5-8 percent of his birth weight during the first week; this is very common. If you are at all concerned about your baby's weight loss, please contact your health care provider. After your baby has regained his birth weight by ten days to two weeks of age, he should gain around 4-7 ounces per week during the first few weeks. Then your baby should gain an average of 1-2 pounds per month during the first six months. From age six months to one year, your little one should gain about 1 pound per month (*The Baby Book, Revised and Updated Edition* 2013, p.150).

Other signs that your baby is thriving are moist skin, lips and inside of mouth. Also, his fontanel, the soft spot on top of his head, should not be depressed. He should latch well and stayed latched on the breast, and have alert times and contentment between feedings. If you are at all concerned if your baby is thriving, please contact your health care provider.

Nutrition for Nursing Mothers

It is important to eat healthfully while breastfeeding, but a perfect diet is not required for an ample milk supply. What should you eat while nursing? According to Dr. William Sears, your daily food plan should include all the healthy foods you normally eat from the five basic food groups, just in greater quantity. Try to choose nutrient-dense selections. Also drink to thirst (*The Baby Book, Revised and Updated Edition 2013*, p.159).

Are there any foods you need to avoid while nursing? Unless you, the mother, have dietary restrictions or you discover that your baby is sensitive or allergic to a particular food, there are no foods you need to avoid. Pregnant women are counseled to avoid certain foods due to increased risk of food-borne illnesses, but these restrictions do not apply to breastfeeding mothers. The only exception I found was that of fish high in mercury. However, both canned light tuna (not albacore) and Pacific wild salmon are two types of fish that can be eaten without restriction.

According to *The Baby Book, Revised and Updated Edition* 2013 (p.167), it is best to limit alcoholic consumption to that once-in-a-while, special occasion drink. If you do decide to have an alcoholic drink, nurse your baby first and then have your glass of wine or beer; that way the alcohol will peak in your bloodstream before your next nursing session, and your baby will get very little, if any, alcohol through your breast milk. The concentration of alcohol is greatest in your milk about 60-90 minutes after you drink it (with food), and then quickly decreases. Therefore, waiting 2-3 hours until the next nursing session will help ensure your breast milk has as little alcohol as possible (*The Baby Book, Revised and Updated Edition 2013*, p.167).

What effect does exercise have on breast milk? Exercise is a great way to slim down after birth, relieve stress and add to your general health and well-being. If you exercise strenuously and then nurse your baby soon afterwards, your milk may have a slightly different taste due to lactic acid build up in your milk. Your baby may or may not notice the taste difference, but it is perfectly fine for baby to drink. One option to avoid the altered taste is to nurse baby first and then exercise. Moderate exercise should not affect the taste of your breast milk.

Starting Solids/Baby-Led Weaning

The American Academy of Pediatrics (AAP), The World Health Organization (WHO), The Canadian Paediatric Society, and the United Kingdom's Minister for Public Health all recommend that babies be exclusively breastfed until six months of age. At six months of age, babies have built up ample levels of enzymes for breaking down solid foods and their intestines are well sealed against allergens (*The Baby Book, Revised and Updated Edition 2013*, p. 228-229). Other signs that your baby is ready for solid food include being able to sit upright, imitating chewing motions, trying to grab food out of your hand, and following your food with his eyes

If your baby is six months or older and is ready for solids, you do not actually need to puree all his food. Pediatricians recommend pureed baby food, because in the past they suggested rice cereal at age two months. A two month old is unable to chew foods that aren't pureed, but an older baby can use his gums and tooth (if he has one) to mash up his food enough to swallow it. You could start with a piece of banana that your baby can hold in his hand and gnaw or mash the banana with a fork and spoon feed it to him. Some moms like to give their babies some mashed avocado, because it not only contains vitamins but lots of fat, too.

Recent studies have shown that it is not necessary to wait a week in-between each new food. Unless there is a family history of food allergies, you can offer new foods more quickly than that (*The Baby Book, Revised and Updated Edition 2013*, p.234).

Medications and Breastfeeding

Most medications are compatible with breastfeeding; there are very few that are not. If you need to take a medication, be sure to let your health care provider know how important breastfeeding is to you and your baby. He or she may be able to find an alternative that is safe to take while breastfeeding. With less compatible medications, you may be able to nurse first and then take it, nurse part time, or take it while nursing an older child even though it may be incompatible while nursing a younger baby. Many lactation consultants have a copy of *Medications and Mother's Milk* by Dr. Hale and can provide info about a medication you are considering taking (*The Baby Book, Revised and Updated Edition*, p.165). Another great resource is the InfantRisk Center, begun by Dr. Hale, for medication questions related to pregnancy and breastfeeding. The phone number is: (806)-352-2519 CST. One other resource, particularly for those middle-of-the-night medication concerns, is Lactmed, an online drug database.

Chapter 2: Common Breastfeeding Concerns

Sore Nipples

Sore nipples are a common occurrence in new breastfeeding mothers. After never having breastfed a baby, suddenly you are nursing almost constantly. The good news is that after a period of adjustment, breastfeeding becomes much more comfortable. Most women find breastfeeding to be easy and enjoyable once the breastfeeding relationship is well established. Those newborn days can sometimes be tough. However, the rewards of continued nursing are substantial for both you and your baby, so hang in there!

If you find yourself with sore nipples, there are some things you can do to improve the situation. First, make sure your baby's mouth is open widely when nursing. If his latch is shallow, and anytime it really hurts, use your clean pinky finger to gently break the suction and try again. The baby should have a good portion of your areola in his mouth - not just the nipple. Also, shooting for an asymmetrical latch - where the baby takes in a larger portion of your breast with his lower jaw - is helpful for a comfortable latch.

Be sure that your baby is tummy to tummy with you and that he doesn't need to turn his head to nurse. You can also try alternative breastfeeding positions if you are still experiencing discomfort. Here are some options: cradle hold (baby is in crook of one arm and the other arm supports his back), cross-cradle hold (baby nurses on one side but the opposite hand supports his head), clutch hold, side-lying nursing, and laid back nursing (nursing in a reclined position with baby on your chest or cradled by your arm). See "Latch and Positioning" in the previous chapter for more information.

Besides poor latch and positioning, another possible cause of nipple soreness is nipple and/or breast injury during a previous nursing session. If this is the case, it does take some time for cracked or bleeding nipples to heal. You can hand express some of your milk and let it dry on your nipple. Your milk is so amazing – it has anti-inflammatory and anti-bacterial properties too! Mild soap and water on your nipple will help reduce the chance of infection.

In terms of comfort measures, pure lanolin is very soothing on nipple abrasions and does not need to be washed off before nursing your baby. Many mothers find hydrogels soothing, and regularly washed and dried breast shells worn occasionally between daytime nursings can help protect sensitive nipples. Going without a bra at home may help ease your discomfort, too (*The Baby Book, Revised and Updated Edition 2013*, p.148-149).

In the long run, keeping the baby latched and positioned well is the best prevention and treatment for sore nipples. If after trying the above strategies, breastfeeding is still painful, not just a little sore or uncomfortable, you may consider calling a lactation consultant or a trained breastfeeding counselor. It is possible that thrush, mastitis or tongue-tie could be causing your nipple soreness, and if so, you may need their help.

Thrush

Thrush is a yeast infection involving the breast. Sometimes mothers contract thrush after having had a vaginal yeast infection and/or taking antibiotics. If you have a vaginal yeast infection at the time of your baby's birth, there is a chance your baby might get thrush during the process of birth. If you've had antibiotics during birth for Group B strep, or after a cesarean section, you and/or your baby may be at higher risk for developing thrush, as well.

If your baby has thrush, he may have a yeasty-smelling diaper rash and/or white spots in his mouth. Symptoms of thrush in the mother include a stabbing, shooting or burning pain in the breast while nursing or even between nursing sessions. The nipples may be pinkish or reddish, and may have flaky skin (*The Baby Book, Revised and Updated Edition 2013*, p. 106-107).

There are many different treatment options for thrush. Limiting sugar and simple carbs such as white flour and white rice in the diet is the easiest first step to take. Also, be sure to eat a nutrient-dense diet as you heal. Dr. William Sears suggests taking an acidophilus supplement daily. Similarly, the acidophilus capsule can be opened and then the contents mixed with water and applied to the baby's mouth. Be sure to wash your nursing bras and pads and anything the baby may suck on in hot, soapy water in between uses. Gentian violet is a non-prescription, topical medication that can be applied to your nipples and the baby's mouth once per day for three or four days to treat thrush. Although effective, some women prefer not to use this particular home remedy, because it is made from coal tar. As always, please consult your health care provider before use.

If over-the-counter treatments do not work, your health care provider can prescribe an anti-fungal medication. Thrush can be transmitted between husband and wife, usually during intercourse, and re-infection can occur in some cases if all three people – mom, dad, and baby - are not treated simultaneously. However, not all thrush cases are this troublesome. If you continue to have symptoms after treatment, please consult a local breastfeeding counselor or your health care provider. It is possible that the problem could be a bacterial infection inside the breast, because the symptoms are the same as thrush. In that case, antibiotics may be necessary (*The Baby Book, Revised and Updated Edition 2013*, p.106-107).

Engorgement

Engorgement is having too much fluid in your breasts. Sometimes women experience engorgement once their milk comes in during the first few days postpartum. IV fluids during labor and birth can also contribute to engorgement. Mothers of babies who suddenly sleep through the night may have engorged breasts upon waking. Engorgement can make it more difficult for the baby to latch onto the breast and can be very uncomfortable for the lactating mother.

By nursing your baby on demand, expressing, making sure your latch and positioning are correct, and avoiding artificial nipples, you help prevent engorgement (*The Baby Book, Revised and Updated Edition 2013*, p.154-155). Actually, just by practicing the Seven Standards of Ecological Breastfeeding (chapter 3), you will be less likely to experience engorged breasts and other problems.

There are several things you can try to relieve engorgement. Hand expressing or pumping just long enough to soften the breast will help make latching easier. Cold compresses may help reduce the inflammation of the breast tissue (*The Baby Book, Revised and Updated* Edition

2013, p. 154-155). Also, some women apply chilled, raw green cabbage leaves to their breasts (avoiding the nipple area) to reduce engorgement. If you do try the cabbage leaf technique, limit the practice to the minimum necessary so baby can latch. If cabbage leaves are applied too often, they can reduce milk supply.

Your doctor may also recommend an anti-inflammatory medication for engorgement.

Plugged Ducts

A plugged duct is an area on the breast that may be tender, red and/or hard. It can be the size of a quarter or even several inches in diameter. Plugged ducts often result from the breasts not being emptied often such as when a baby starts sleeping through the night. Pressure from a baby carrier or underwire bra can also sometimes contribute to plugged ducts.

If left untreated, a plugged duct can turn into mastitis, so it is best to treat it as soon as possible. If you believe you have a plugged duct, massage and apply warm compresses to the affected area while breastfeeding your baby. Continue breastfeeding often on both breasts so that your breasts will be emptied regularly, and point your baby's chin in the direction of the plugged duct. Some women breastfeed on the affected breast first at each nursing session while there is a plugged duct to make sure it is being emptied as much as possible. If you think your bra may be to blame, try a different bra or go without a bra for a few days. If you have plugged ducts often, eating eggs (which contain lecithin) may help prevent them in the future. If the plugged duct does not go away and you experience flu like symptoms, redness radiating out from the area and/or pain, please consult with your health care provider (*The Baby Book, Revised and Updated Edition 2013*, p.155).

Mastitis

Mastitis is an infection, or simply an inflammation, of the breast. Symptoms include a warm, red, sensitive area on the breast, possibly a fever, chills, and flu-like symptoms. Mastitis often occurs when nipple damage allows the entry of bacteria into the breast, the breasts are not emptied as often as necessary, there is pressure from an underwire bra or something else, or the body isn't getting enough rest. It may begin with a plugged duct or it may not (*The Baby Book, Revised and Updated Edition 2013*, p.155).

The first treatment is lots of rest and ample breast drainage. Keep the affected breast as empty as possible but continue breastfeeding on the other side regularly, too. Try the comfort measures listed in the engorgement section, and you can also take an over the counter pain reliever/anti-inflammatory if your health care provider approves. If you are not getting worse, keep treating yourself at home for 24 hours. Also, consider not wearing a bra and gently massaging your affected breast several times per day. If home treatment does not improve your condition, call your health care provider; he or she may give you an antibiotic. There are many antibiotics compatible with breastfeeding; let your health care provider know that you do not want to interrupt breastfeeding. Breastfeeding is still best for you and your baby, even if you are feeling ill or have an infection (*The Baby Book, Revised and Updated Edition 2013*, p.155)

Increasing Your Milk Supply

There may be times when your once adequate milk supply seems to be less abundant than usual. Sometimes a baby nurses less during sickness or during a long road trip and your milk supply drops. Maybe it is the holiday season and you have been more preoccupied than usual and nursing less.

The best way to increase your supply during those temporary lags is to nurse more often. Some mothers take a day to just lie in bed, read, rest and NURSE. Do lots of skin to skin time with your baby and offer the breast often. When the breast is emptied often, the brain gets the message to make more milk.

If your supply is still not quite where it should be after nursing more often, pumping with a breast pump or hand expressing your milk will give your breasts some added stimulation. Eating certain foods like oatmeal, barley, and brown rice may also help increase your supply. The herb, fenugreek, is effective for increasing milk supply in many women. As with any herb or medication, please consult your health care provider before consuming. Fenugreek, in particular, can lower blood sugar levels, which can be a concern in those taking insulin. Also, avoid herbs and medications that decrease milk supply such as parsley, sage, and peppermint (*The Baby Book, Revised and Updated Edition 2013*, p.152-154).

If your supply is still low after following the above suggestions, consider calling a lactation consultant.

Oversupply

Having an over-abundance of milk may appear to some to be a problem they would love to have. However, it can be frustrating and uncomfortable for both mom and baby.

Some symptoms of oversupply in the baby include: repeatedly coming off the breast and/or arching after your milk lets down, spitting up and needing to burp often, not wanting to nurse to sleep or just for comfort, green and mucousy stools, gassiness, faster than usual weight gain, and diaper rash (*The Baby Book, Revised and Updated Edition 2013*, p.404-405).

If you have an oversupply problem, there are several things you can try to help balance your supply. First, try nursing only on one side for each feed. If you feel exceptionally full on the other side, offer that breast for a short time just to soften it. If you are still too full after nursing on one side per feeding, consider block nursing. This means that for say the next two hours, you will only nurse your baby on the left side. Then, for the next two hours, you will only nurse your baby on the right side. More emphasis should be on your comfort level and amount of fullness rather than how much time has elapsed. Another possibility is to try different nursing positions such as laid-back nursing (nursing in a reclined position with baby on your chest) or nursing while lying down. Also, you might try consuming the herb, sage, which decreases milk supply.

Breast Refusal

Sometimes a baby that nurses well and is not close to weaning age suddenly rejects the breast for part of a day or even a few days. This can be very nerve-racking for mom and baby, too. There are many possible reasons for a nursing strike such as illness in the baby, teething, stress in the family, and even something minor like a different deodorant for mom.

Sometimes encouraging baby to return to nursing requires creativity and lots of patience. Try to stay calm. Attempt to breastfeed your baby when he is content or sleepy. Hold your baby close to you, skin to skin, without a shirt or while taking a relaxing bath. Sing to him or rock him.

In the meantime, especially if your baby refuses to nurse for a day or longer, he will be hungry and still need milk. You can hand express or pump your breast milk and give it in a small cup or even an eye dropper. If the situation does not resolve quickly in a day or two, please call your doctor, local breastfeeding counselor or a lactation consultant for more assistance (*The Baby Book, Revised and Updated Edition 2013*, p.188-189).

Chapter 3: Ecological Breastfeeding

Dr. William Sears, pediatrician and author, was asked about the key to successful breastfeeding and responded, "Frequency, frequency, frequency." That is also a summary of ecological breastfeeding. Ecological breastfeeding is the human biological norm, the way breastfeeding is supposed to take place in nature. Mother and baby stay close to each other. The mother is in tune to her baby and nurses him when is hungry, upset, tired or when he just needs to suckle or to feel close to her. She nurses him during his nap time and during the night. This special dance between mom and baby helps the child gradually grow more independent as he is ready, and provides many health benefits to both mother and baby as were previously mentioned. Also, there is a special side effect to ecological breastfeeding - infertility - which is nature's way of spacing families.

The Secret of Natural Mothering
by Maureen Armendariz

So often, when a young mother hears about Ecological Breastfeeding, her mind jumps to "the cost." You know, what it will cost her - sharing her bed, turning down certain party invitations, being always 'on', and maybe the worry about how long it will go on. A mother, whether choosing eco-breastfeeding or not, does give a lot. And our society ill prepares parents for that fact.

But what a mother gives to her naturally-mothered child is only half the equation. No - it is less than half the equation. Because what can't be properly communicated before it is experienced, is what an Ecologically Breastfed child gives back.

You give yourself to your baby unreservedly; he gives you an adoration you have to feel to believe. You give your baby your arms and breasts when he is sad, hungry, frightened, or hurt; he gives you a sense of empowerment - a sure knowledge that you and you alone are the most important being in the universe to him. You give your baby a place in your bed; he gives you hundreds of peaceful nights.

My husband and I have the privilege of knowing a wonderful Catholic psychologist. Several years ago he was working on his thesis; attachment disorder was his subject. He was talking with us about cosleeping and bedsharing. He was wondering how it worked for us, how we felt about all the sacrificed sleep. We looked at each other and burst out laughing. "Well, Doctor, we can't answer that question, since we don't sacrifice any sleep!" He was surprised, and delighted. Studies do show that while bedsharing mothers do wake more often than their crib-using counterparts, the bedsharing moms report feeling better-rested. Most bedsharing mothers are back to sleep before the milk even lets down!

So often what looks like a sacrifice for the greater good of our children turns out to be a greater blessing to us than we could have fathomed. It's actually a simple Christian concept of spirituality. The more we embrace a sacrifice, the sweeter it becomes, until it ceases to be a sacrifice and becomes, in the end, a treasure we would not trade.

And that, to me, is the secret of natural mothering.

The Seven Standards of Ecological Breastfeeding

Ecological breastfeeding is the oldest form of natural child spacing. It involves not just exclusive breastfeeding but also a special lifestyle of breastfeeding. This way of mothering is very natural; although it must be acknowledged that Western culture and values generally do not support the practice of full ecological breastfeeding. Today the practice of ecological breastfeeding is considered counter-cultural. The Catholic Nursing Mothers League, while recognizing any amount of breastfeeding is valuable, encourages all mothers to consider practicing full ecological breastfeeding. The best explanation of ecological breastfeeding can be found in the classic work, *Breastfeeding and Natural Child Spacing*, by Catholic author, Sheila Kippley. In it, she introduces and explains the seven standards that comprise this practice:

1. Breastfeed exclusively for the first six months of life.
2. Pacify or comfort your baby at your breasts.
3. Don't use bottles or pacifiers.
4. Sleep with your baby for night feedings.
5. Sleep with your baby for daily nap feedings.
6. Nurse frequently day and night and avoid schedules.
7. Avoid any practice that restricts nursing or separates you from your baby.

(*Breastfeeding and Natural Child Spacing 2008*, p. 168)

Standard 1: Breastfeed exclusively for the first six months

Exclusive breastfeeding means that no other food or liquid - even water - is given in addition to nursing at the breast.

This standard is supported by the American Academy of Pediatrics, the World Health Organization, and most major health organizations. The newest research actually shows that waiting until at least six months before offering solid food is best for baby's health. Babies often get their first tooth and are starting to sit up unassisted at around six months old, so it seems waiting until six months is the way nature intended. Also, following nature is one way we glorify our Creator.

By waiting to introduce solids until six months, you give your baby's digestive system the necessary amount of time to mature. Also, exclusive breastfeeding encourages the growth of all the wonderful probiotics your baby needs. Researchers looked at the guts of formula-fed babies versus exclusively breastfed babies and found a distinctive difference between the types of bacteria that colonized each baby's gut (*The Baby Book, Revised and Updated Edition 2013*, p.212).

Sometimes a new mother cannot imagine breastfeeding for so long. However, once the breastfeeding relationship is well established around six weeks of age, nursing often becomes easier and more enjoyable. These same women who couldn't imagine nursing until six months often cannot imagine stopping once the six month mark arrives!

Standard 2: Pacify or comfort your baby at the breast

Babies have a physiological need to suck. They often even suck their fingers and thumbs in the womb. Artificial pacifiers were designed to satisfy a baby's sucking needs and to make mothers' lives easier. However, nature has a better way. By pacifying your baby often at your breast, you help stimulate a good milk supply and increase the amount of time of closeness and love between you and your baby. This extra stimulation from comforting your baby at your breast is one main difference between exclusive breastfeeding and ecological breastfeeding. You can exclusively breastfeed yet use pacifiers or other soothers and only nurse your baby when he is hungry - not for comfort. However, ecological breastfeeding includes nursing for comfort and pacification and often leads to several months or years of natural infertility.

Many babies love the comfort of nursing to sleep, and many older babies nurse to be close to mom. Toddlers who get hurt or who feel overwhelmed often nurse to feel right with the world again. It is such an easy way to help a child feel better! Nursing during or just after immunizations or other medical procedures can reduce your child's pain. The hormones that calm a baby also calm you, too, so it is a win-win situation.

Some moms wonder if it is really possible not to use pacifiers at all. I, personally, have never used pacifiers with any of my babies. My babies do enjoy nursing often, but even with several older children for whom to care, I still have a few moments to sit down and nurse my youngest. Part of this very book was written while nursing a baby!

Research has shown that by avoiding pacifiers and artificial teats, your baby's jaw has a better chance of developing correctly which translates into less risk of needing orthodontic work in the future. Breastfeeding without pacifiers also reduces thumbsucking, leads to better speech, and contributes to a longer duration of breastfeeding (*The Seven Standards of Ecological Breastfeeding*, p. 10).

The American Academy of Pediatrics (AAP) recommends pacifier use at night (after breastfeeding is well established) to reduce the incidence of sudden infant death syndrome (SIDS). However, Dr. James McKenna and Dr. William Sears among others have concluded that safe bedsharing and breastfeeding are excellent ways to reduce SIDS risk without needing to introduce a pacifier. After all, an artificial pacifier is just replacing the non-nutritive suckling that naturally would occur at the breast (*The Baby Book, Revised and Updated Edition* 2013, p.120, 122).

Standard 3: Don't use bottles or pacifiers

A baby nursing directly at the breast provides the strongest stimulation for a good milk supply and for natural lactational amenorrhea and infertility. Plus, by avoiding bottles and pacifiers your baby avoids the possibility of nipple confusion during the first few weeks of life. As Catholics we are called to be good stewards of the earth. Ecologically breastfeeding without bottles and pacifiers helps reduce the amount of plastics in the landfills. So, in actuality, you are contributing to a good milk supply, avoiding some breastfeeding difficulties, naturally spacing your family and taking care of the earth! And you thought you were just simply nursing your baby!

But is ecological breastfeeding without the use of bottles and pacifiers practical? From personal experience, I emphatically say "yes!" I have breastfed all my children and have never needed to use bottles or pacifiers. As part of the natural mothering lifestyle, I just simply take my young nursling with me when I go grocery shopping, on retreat with the Holy Family Institute, to the library with my older children, and to an occasional movie in the theaters to just name a few. I have even taken a nursing baby on my weekly evening out "by myself" and on date night with my husband. I have several children so just taking the quiet, nursing baby on my night out still refreshes me from the challenging work of motherhood. My husband and I also have a chance to have some needed quiet time on date night while we hold the baby and enjoy a good meal at a restaurant.

What if your baby's grandparents want to feed him a bottle? Offer them other ways to bond with the baby or to help care for him such as diaper changes, rocking him to sleep after he is done nursing, playing with him, or bathing him. Also, let the grandparents know that when he starts solids, they can help spoon feed him or can sit him on their lap during dinner.

Many moms also enjoy wearing their babies in slings or baby carriers. This enables the mother to do some work around the house or to help other children with their needs while satisfying the baby's need to be close to mom. You can breastfeed your baby in many of today's slings, too. When you purchase a sling, it usually comes with an instructional booklet and/or DVD if you would like to learn how to do this. Also, ask at your church's nursing mothers group meeting for additional assistance.

Standard 4: Sleep with your baby for night feedings

Although the American Academy of Pediatrics discourages bedsharing, some experts such as Dr. James McKenna and infant sleep researcher and author, think bedsharing can be done safely and that it has many benefits to both mom and baby. Dr. James McKenna's sleep studies show moms curling themselves in a protective manner around their babies as they sleep. Also, their sleep cycles often synchronize so closely so that the moms wake up moments before their babies start to stir. This special awareness mothers have of their babies reduces the risk of SIDS (*The Baby Book, Revised and Updated Edition 2013*, p.120-122).

By nursing a few times at night, which bedsharing babies tend to do, your milk supply is stimulated. Many babies actually take in a large portion of their daily calories during those nighttime nursings. Breast stimulation at night contributes more to lactational amenorrhea than the same number of nursings during the day. Some moms do not start ovulating and cycling again until their babies do not need to nurse anymore at night.

If you are a new mom or even a mom of more than one child, you know how exhausting nighttime parenting can be at times. The nice aspect of breastfeeding is that it minimizes the times you need to get out of bed and even wake up completely. Ask a mom who breastfeeds and bedshares just how many times the baby wakes to nurse. She very well may tell you she has no idea!

How lovely it is for both mom and baby (and dad, too!) when all the baby has to do is stir a little bit and the mom half wakes up, latches the baby on and all go back to sleep (dad probably never even heard the baby at all). The alternative to breastfeeding and co-sleeping is to get up out of your warm bed and make a bottle of formula in the kitchen. Then, if you follow the World Health Organization guidelines, you will need to first boil the water to kill possible pathogens present before mixing it with powdered or concentrated formula. Latching baby on and going back to sleep in 30 seconds sounds a lot more appealing!

Characteristics of a safe bedsharing surface include:

- Having a firm mattress with no gaps at the head and foot boards
- tight fitting sheets
- light blankets instead of heavy ones
- no pillows near baby's face

Please do NOT bedshare if:

- either you or your husband smokes at all; smoking is one of the biggest risk factors for SIDS
- you or your spouse are intoxicated, on sleep inducing medication, or very tired
- your baby is under the age of one years old and there are other children or pets in your bed; older children are not as aware of the baby while sleeping as you are
- the bed contains soft bedding, pillows, gaps between the mattress and bed frame or wall or bedrail

Also, dressing your baby in heavy clothing, putting your baby to sleep on his stomach, swaddling him, and sleeping with your baby on a couch all increase the risks of harm to your baby (*The Baby Book, Revised and Updated Edition 2013*, p.350-351).

On a personal note, a king-size bed has made bedsharing so much more comfortable for us, especially as each baby becomes a toddler. Toddlers tend to sleep in unusual positions and sometimes take up more room than Mom and Dad! I also know some couples who sleep with their baby on a mattress on the floor; we did this with our first for part of the first year. Be creative and design your own special safe bedsharing area.

What about marital intimacy while bedsharing? This is another area where creativity comes into play. If your baby is young, you could put him in a little bassinet on the floor. If he is older, a crib or toddler bed mattress on the floor works well, too. You and your husband can also spend some couple time in a spare room or guest room in your house after your baby goes to sleep for the night. Just remember to think outside the box and find what works for you and your husband!

Standard 5: Sleep with baby for a daily nap feeding

Either relaxing or sleeping while your baby nurses to sleep for an afternoon nap is a wonderful way to get yourself some much needed rest. Babies often enjoy nursing for part of their nap or all of their nap. We live in such a busy society that it is very tempting to fit in as much as we can each day. However, nature has other ideas. I don't know about you, but I find there is a lull in the middle to late afternoon when I feel tired and need a snack and some quiet time before I need to make dinner. Oftentimes this is when my baby wants to nurse and nap too. By going along with this natural tendency, you also allow for more stimulation at the breast which can lengthen your time of lactation amenorrhea. Sheila Kippley recommends at least one nap nursing for 30 minutes each day. Based on her experience with breastfeeding moms, missing the nap can be a key factor in the early return of fertility (*The Seven Standards of Ecological Breastfeeding*, p. 41-42).

If you have older children, you could incorporate a family rest time when baby is sleeping. All the children can sleep, look at books quietly, or watch a short DVD during this time. If you, yourself, just plan to rest during baby's nap and not actually fall asleep, you could have a basket of picture books, quiet toys or books on CD for you to share with your other children to keep them entertained.

If a mother calls me about a plugged duct or possible symptoms of mastitis, one of the first suggestions I give is REST. I know that mothers have a lot of responsibilities and many do not live close to extended family members. However, we need to allow ourselves time for rest and recreation. Remember that God created everything in six days and rested on the seventh; if God rested, so should we. Jesus was asleep on the boat the afternoon of the big storm. Jesus also ate and drank and rested with friends during various times in the Gospels. When I am well rested, I am more patient with my children and do not feel as overwhelmed by the chaos of my family. Now I should go heed my own advice ☺

Standard 6: Nurse Frequently Day and Night and avoid schedules

Babies were designed to nurse many times per day. Human milk is low in fat and also digests quickly, requiring frequent nursing sessions. Milk production works according to supply and demand; the more you nurse, the more milk you make. There are women who cannot produce enough milk even when breastfeeding often due to insufficient breast tissue, hormonal imbalances, and relactation for adoptive nursing. However, these are rare situations; only 5% of women cannot physically breastfeed.

One physiological reason not to schedule feedings is that every woman has a different breast storage capacity. Women with a smaller breast storage capacity will end up nursing their baby more often if they follow their baby's lead. Storage capacity is not necessarily related to breast size.

Another reason not to schedule nursing is that you will not know when your baby needs your milk supply to increase during a growth spurt. If you have an older child, you know there are times when he needs more to eat, especially adolescent boys. They can go through periods of time when they are simply ravenous. After several days or even a week, it seems to pass and they are back to their normal eating habits. We, as adults, also desire more or less food sometimes due to exercise, sickness, stress, etc. Why would a baby be any different?

Several researchers have studied the effect of breastfeeding on fertility. One such researcher, Dr. James Wood of the University of Michigan's Population Studies Center, studied the Gainj people of New Guinea to determine the effect of breastfeeding on their childbirth rates. Gainj mothers tend to breastfeed their children frequently but in shorter spurts. The mothers in the study breastfed their babies on average every 24 minutes and their three year olds on average every 80 minutes. The interval between nursings very slowly lengthened, and this was found to be significant for delaying the return of fertility. The Gainj people have an average family size of 4.3 children, and an average of 44 months between births. They do not practice contraception or abortion (*The Seven Standards of Ecological Breastfeeding*, p. 46).

Also, Konner and Worthman studied the !Kung tribe in southern Africa. The mothers had an average of 44 months between births and did not practice contraception. The !Kung mothers keep their children under two years old close to them during the day and night, and the children nurse often – a few times per hour for just a few minutes at a time. The frequency of suckling seems to be the key to their natural infertility, also (*The Seven Standards of Ecological Breastfeeding*, p. 47).

Another researcher, Dr. R.V. Short, studied the !Kung in southern Africa and a Papua New Guinea tribe and theorized that it is the biochemical composition of human breast milk - low in fat, protein and dry matter - that helps explain the frequency of a child's suckling. He noted that gorillas suckle several times per hour, sleep with their babies, and have four to five year birth intervals just like the other tribes mentioned. He also states that it is the frequency of breastfeeding that is most important in the natural infertility of breastfeeding. (*The Seven Standards of Ecological Breastfeeding*, p. 47).

Lastly, Dr. H. William Taylor studied a group of American mothers who breastfed similarly to the above stated tribes; their average time of natural infertility was 14 months. He found that the mothers who nursed their babies for less time per session but more often tended to ovulate later than those who nursed for longer sessions but less frequently (*The Seven Standards of Ecological Breastfeeding*, p. 47). All of the above explains the subtitle of Sheila Kippley's book I've been referencing – The Frequency Factor.

Standard 7: Avoid any practice that restricts nursing or separates you from your baby

Mothers and babies are biologically programmed to want and to need to be together; that is why they are often described as a mother baby dyad. Current research shows that your presence is especially important in your baby's first three years of life. You help your baby learn to trust you and to feel secure and safe by breastfeeding him and by staying close to him. This close relationship also contributes to optimal brain growth and emotional development (*The Seven Standards of Ecological Breastfeeding*, p. 56).

Once breastfeeding is well established, it is effortless and enjoyable for many women and babies. If you need to go out, why not just bring baby with you? If you feel uncomfortable nursing in public, there are many stylish nursing covers you can buy online. However, nursing covers are not necessary if you feel comfortable without one. You can also use a blanket or a sweater to help you nurse more modestly. Most states have laws in place to help protect a woman's right to breastfeed in public.

Very little equipment is needed when going out with your breastfed baby. All you need is a diaper, some wipes and a change of clothes in case of diaper leakage. Your milk is always warm and ready for your baby to drink. This is especially helpful when taking a longer trip, for instance, in an airplane. There are fewer and fewer items, it seems, that are allowed on one's person when going through security. Breastfeeding just makes it that much easier to navigate that whole process. Also, by comforting your baby at the breast at take-off, landing, and while in the air, you will help make the experience enjoyable for you and your baby.

Once you get used to taking baby everywhere with you, I think it will grow on you and you will feel more and more confident about it. It seems like more work to find someone to watch your baby for a few hours and then pump while you are out, then to simply bring your baby with you. Also, as time goes on, you will learn which businesses have changing tables and chairs for you to sit in and nurse. Some businesses even have toy boxes for older infants and toddlers. It will be a fun adventure to take a day trip with baby!

If you do need a little time out by yourself (I find that I start to come unglued when I do not get at least a short time out once or twice a week), your husband or other family member may be able to assist you. You might want to schedule such a time during one of baby's naptimes or just after nursing him. I like to bring a cell phone with me in case the baby suddenly needs me. Also, adjust your amount of time gone to the age and needs of your baby. Sheila Kippley recommends waiting until your baby is at least one year of age before beginning separations.

The Interconnectedness of the Seven Standards

Notice that many of the Seven Standards are interconnected. If you nurse frequently and avoid pacifiers and schedules, you have a good chance of achieving your goal of exclusive breastfeeding for the first six months. If you avoid separation from your baby and avoid bottles, you will automatically be nursing frequently day and night. If you avoid pacifiers and bottles, you will be comforting your baby at your breast. The design is very cyclical and beautiful if you think about it. The key to the Seven Standards is seeing yourself and your baby as a mother-baby dyad. If you look at it from this perspective, you will choose to stay close to your baby (your baby would always choose to be close to you). If you nurse on demand and are always with your baby, frequent suckling will occur, which lends itself to natural infertility.

The First Three Months Postpartum

Sooner or later your fertility will return. With ecological breastfeeding there is about a seven percent chance of becoming fertile in the first six months, especially in the second three months.

Any vaginal bleeding during the first 56 days postpartum while exclusively or ecologically breastfeeding can be ignored; it does not indicate fertility. That is the consensus of those researching the Lactational Amenorrhea Method (LAM) – exclusive breastfeeding for the first six months (*The Baby Book, Revised and Updated Edition* 2013, p. 158). If you are practicing all Seven Standards of ecological breastfeeding and you have not had any vaginal bleeding during the third month postpartum, your chances of pregnancy are almost zero.

The 4th and 5th Months Postpartum

There is less than a 1% chance of pregnancy if you are following the Seven Standards of ecological breastfeeding and have not had any vaginal bleeding after the first 56 days postpartum.

Six to Eight Months and Beyond

When your baby starts to eat or drink something other than your breast milk (usually sometime around 6-8 months), weaning is actually beginning. If you plan on nursing for an extended period of time, the weaning process will be very gradual and may take months or even years! The possibility of pregnancy before the first menstruation at this time is 6% but can be reduced to 1% by also practicing systematic Natural Family Planning (charting one or several signs of fertility such as mucus, temperature, position of cervix, and hormonal status). Some women will experience many more months of natural infertility, especially if they and their babies gradually reduce the frequency and amount of nursing. Even if you do begin to ovulate again while following all of the Seven Standards but the first one, your cycles may not be fertile for a period of time. Many women (about 70%) experience between 9 and 20 months of breastfeeding amenorrhea when ecologically breastfeeding. The average time for first menstruation is 14-15 months postpartum in the North American culture (*The Seven Standards of Ecological Breastfeeding*, p. 103-104).

Natural Family Planning Resources for Nursing Mothers

At some point, either while still breastfeeding or after weaning, your fertility will return. At first, you may just have patches of mucus days if you were previously dry or you may start experiencing patches of more fertile type mucus against the background of continuous, tacky or sticky type mucus. Then just before your first postpartum ovulation or menses, you will most likely notice lots of mucus. After prayer and discussion, you and your husband may decide you should practice natural family planning to postpone pregnancy.

There are several NFP methods, fortunately, from which to choose. The sympto-thermal method involves observing and charting cervical mucus, temperature, and also the position of the cervix if desired. The most recent scientific study on the method determined its effectiveness to be 99.6% in postponing pregnancy if used according to the rules. NFP International (NFPI) teaches the symptom-thermal method and includes ecological breastfeeding as part of the total NFP package.

There are also a few mucus only methods. The Creighton model uses a standardized system of charting based on sensation when wiping and mucus observed for various characteristics. The Billings Method of Ovulation (BOM) emphasizes sensation during daily activities and the observation of mucus when using the restroom. Women use their own personal language when charting.

The Marquette Method uses the Clearblue Easy Fertility Monitor and possibly mucus to determine the fertile and infertile times. They conducted a study in 2013 specifically with breastfeeding women using only the

Clearblue Easy Fertility Monitor. It was found to have a 98% perfect use effectiveness rate. The advantage of the Marquette Method is the Monitor will evaluate your fertility/infertility in terms of two pre-pregnancy hormones that it detects in your urine. This can be helpful during the transition from non-cycling to cycling. However, the monitor and strips can be expensive.

There are also a few other organizations that teach NFP. Visit the USCCB Directory of NFP Providers to see the complete list.

Should You Wean Your Nursling to Conceive Another Baby?

Is ecological breastfeeding working too well for you in terms of its natural infertility effect? Are you desiring another baby but wonder what is God's will in this matter? First, pray with your spouse about how you are feeling. Try not to compare your family size with that of others. This a private decision between you, your spouse, and God.

Then think about the answers to some of these questions: How old is your nursling? Is he at least one (if not, formula supplementation would be necessary) and maybe even over two years old? The World Health Organization recommends breastfeeding until at least age two and then for longer if mutually desired. However, this does not necessarily mean waiting for two years before seeking pregnancy. How does your child respond when you try to distract him instead of nursing him? If he cries a lot and seems very unhappy, he may not be ready to reduce the amount he nurses. Also, does he eat solid food well? If he still does not eat solids well, he is probably nursing a large part for the nutritional benefits in addition to comfort.

Your milk still has the same great nutritional value it had when your baby was younger. Are you cycling? If you are cycling and just not getting pregnant, keeping an NFP chart may help you conceive. Would you regret having weaned your nursling if you are unable to conceive again in the future? God may have other plans for your family, so you want to make sure weaning is in the best interest of this particular child.

If you do decide weaning is the right decision, it is best to slowly drop one nursing at a time so your child and milk supply gradually adjust. Usually the bedtime and naptime nursings are the most challenging to drop, so maybe choose a time during the day when your child is not tired and is easily distractible. Be sure to offer lots of attention, affection, and snacks. ☺

Nurturing the Marriage Relationship in the Ecological Breastfeeding Family

There are a lot of authors that suggest overnight and weekend getaways as necessary for a healthy marriage. If you practice ecological breastfeeding, however, these trips are not always advisable. When your youngest child weans, maybe a trip like this will be a possibility. What to do in the meantime? My husband and I have a weekly two hour date night. If I have a nursling or a clingy toddler, she comes with us. Otherwise the youngest stays home with her brothers (our oldest son is a teenager). Before our oldest was a teenager, we had a regular babysitter for date night. If you do not have a teenage son or daughter or you cannot afford a sitter, consider trading babysitting with a friend. Another idea is to have a date night at home by putting on a family DVD for the kids and sharing a special meal with your sweetie at the kitchen table.

In our family we have a bedtime for the oldest kids. This way my husband and I have quiet time together in the evening. Our nursing baby is welcome to join us. Once our second child came along, we realized that even if the baby stays up with us, it is still quieter and more conducive to couple time than when all the kids are up. I know some moms who do not have bedtimes. They most likely set aside other times for special couple time, possibly after dad gets home from work. As your children get older, you can let them know that for the first 20 minutes after dad gets home, they need to play or read quietly so that the two of you have some time to reconnect after a busy day.

There are other little ways you and your husband can stay connected while raising children. You can talk on the phone during the day, exchange text messages or emails and have lunch together if your husband is able to come home from work. You may consider asking friends what works for them or subscribing to inspirational blogs for more ideas.

The Importance of Fathers in the Breastfeeding Relationship

Fathers are also very important to the mom-baby breastfeeding relationship. Dad has a unique role to play - supporter of the mother and the family. He is so essential to the breastfeeding relationship that the Catholic Nursing Mothers League acknowledges his importance in its principles (chapter 6).

I know that some new dads feel left out at first, because their wives are breastfeeding. However, there is a lot he can do to support you, the mother, physically, emotionally and spiritually. He can bring you something to eat and drink when you are nursing your baby or are resting. He can help with household chores. He can listen to you talk about whatever is on your mind and give lots of hugs and kisses, especially if you are feeling overwhelmed or experiencing the baby blues. Last, but not least, your husband can pray for you and lead the other children in prayer as spiritual head of the family.

In terms of helping with the baby, your husband can change diapers, give baths, burp the baby, rock baby to sleep, play with the baby and carry him in a sling. He can also hold baby on his bare chest for lots of skin to skin contact. Babies usually like this a lot - at least mine have. If mom needs assistance from a trained breastfeeding counselor or lactation consultant, he can be the go between, so mom can rest. Dads are special and very much needed!

Gentle Parenting

What exactly does this entail? Well, when your child is young and you are still nursing him, it can mean practicing the ecological breastfeeding and natural mothering lifestyle. As your child grows older, it represents a mothering/parenting philosophy of enjoying your child(ren)'s presence and gently guiding him through conversation and instruction, active participation in the Mass and sacraments, and sometimes more firm but still loving guidance.

Mary and Joseph were the ideal example of "gentle parents" beginning with Mary nursing Jesus for most likely four years, according to Fr. Rob Jack at the Bible Institute, Xavier University. They celebrated religious feasts together as a family and spent time talking to each other. When Jesus was 12 years old and lost for a few days on the way back from the Passover celebration, Mary and Joseph were very worried, of course, but they responded gently.

"The Prodigal Son" parable in the Gospels teaches parents how to respond to a child that goes astray. The son squandered his inheritance but eventually realized the immorality of his ways. He made things right with his father, and his father embraced him with joy. This symbolizes how our Father in heaven responds to us when we stray and return. The brother of the prodigal son was probably expecting his father to punish his brother but that is not what happened. The prodigal son had already experienced the consequences of his poor actions – needing to take care of "unclean" pigs and being hungry. What he needed next was forgiveness.

Relationship work can be very challenging! It involves being sensitive to what is important to your husband and children, being flexible, modifying our expectations at times of our family members and ourselves, and forgiving often. We all make mistakes and have regrets, but St. Paul urges us to persevere and finish the race. Even if our own childhood and relationship history were far from ideal, we can look to the Gospels, 2 Corinthians 13 and St. Therese of Lisieux for guidance.

Have you been searching for THE instruction book on how to raise your children? There really isn't a book that will tell you how to handle every situation and fix every flaw in yourself and in your child. However, there are two Catholic parenting books that come close: *Parenting with Grace* by the Popcaks and *The Discipline Book* by Dr. and Mrs. Sears.

Even though it is best not to overuse parenting techniques, it may be helpful to you to have a few basic discipline strategies for those trying days of parenting. Do-overs are wonderful ways to teach your child the correct way to behave. If your child speaks disrespectfully to you or calls his sibling a name, ask him to "do it over."

Natural consequences are those consequences that result without your intervention. For example, if your child leaves his new bike outside in the rain and it gets stolen or it rusts, he will experience the results of his actions without you needing to do anything. If your elementary school age child plays in the mud and then tracks mud onto the carpet in the house, a "logical consequence" for doing so would be to vacuum the carpet. Sometimes you may need to restrict your child's privileges when they misbehave or will not listen even after you have told them what is expected.

Time-outs for YOU can be critical on some days. If you feel like you are about to lose your cool, you may consider spending ten minutes alone in your bedroom to calm down and to decide what to do next. If your child is highly emotional, he may need some cool down time away from you and other people. Separation of two siblings is sometimes necessary when they refuse to be nice to each other or if one child is physically or verbally hurting another child.

Helping kids transition from one activity to another by giving them a five or ten minute warning helps them feel like you find their activities important. Counting to three to get your children moving more quickly in the right direction can be useful especially if you have to get to a doctor's appointment or Mass on time.

As time goes on, you will develop your own unique parenting style. Do your best to be responsive to your child. Ask the Holy Spirit to guide you and then quietly listen for the answer. Also, ask the Holy Spirit for confidence in yourself and remember that you are the expert on how to parent your child!

Chapter 4: Catholic Motherhood

Breastfeeding and Church Tradition

It may pleasantly surprise you that the Catholic Church has a long-standing tradition in support of breastfeeding. The Church, first of all, follows natural law. What could be more natural and in tune with God's plan for humans than feeding your baby the milk your own body produces? Ecological breastfeeding, too, follows natural law. You follow your baby's needs for milk and comfort using the body God gave you as a gift. You are then a gift to your child. The infertility that results is nature's design and another gift to you.

As I write this, there is a heated debate taking place on a popular Catholic internet site. They are discussing whether or not breastfeeding can be done in a selfish manner due to its natural benefit of infertility. My personal opinion is "no." You can't force your baby to nurse if he doesn't want to. Even if you wake him in the middle of the night to nurse in the hopes of extending your own natural infertility, he will only nurse if he needs it. On a personal note, I have bedshared with all my children, and they woke naturally one to several times per night until around age two without any help from me. Also, in the over ten years I have been involved with supporting nursing mothers, no one has mentioned that they wake their baby to nurse during the night (except for maybe a sleepy newborn baby in the first week of life)! On the contrary, moms usually accept this phase of life and all it entails or try different techniques to get their babies to sleep through the night. Then there is also the situation of many women who would love to have another baby but are unable to conceive because they are breastfeeding.

In terms of support from popes and bishops, Pope Gregory the Great, Pope Benedict XIV, Pope Pius XII, and (Saint) Pope John Paul II all showed support of breastfeeding. The two latter popes publicly spoke to mothers about its importance (*Breastfeeding and Catholic Motherhood*, p. 32-34). The current pope, Pope Francis, has been especially supportive of breastfeeding moms. On Holy Thursday, he washed the feet of twelve pregnant and nursing moms - one mom was actively nursing her baby during the actual washing of feet! On another occasion, he encouraged mothers to nurse their hungry babies during a baptism ceremony in the Sistine Chapel. At least two bishops also advocated for breastfeeding - Bishop James T. McHugh and Alfonso Cardinal Lopez Trujillo. (*Breastfeeding and Catholic Motherhood*, p.36-37). As you can see, the Magisterium wholeheartedly supports nursing moms and babies.

Several priests actively promote breastfeeding in their own unique ways. Father Virtue wrote a chapter on breastfeeding in his doctoral dissertation, *Mother and Infant*. Father Timothy Sauppe created a Madonna chapel and developed a rosary of five mysteries in honor of Mary's breastfeeding relationship with Jesus which was granted an imprimatur (*Breastfeeding and Catholic Motherhood*, p. 38-40). I am sure there are countless other Church leaders who are doing a wonderful job supporting nursing mothers.

Christian artwork often portrays Mary breastfeeding Jesus, sometimes with her breast exposed. Scripture mentions breastfeeding no less than 12 times, and weaning is often mentioned as taking place at the end of the second or third year of life.

The Catholic Church honors two souls in heaven as patron saints of breastfeeding. St. Giles is one of the official patron saints of breastfeeding mothers. He was a hermit in Southern France in the late 600s - early 700s who reportedly sustained himself for several years only on the milk of a hind. His feast day is September 1. In addition, the diocese of St. Augustine, FL celebrates the feast of Our Lady of La Leche on Oct. 11. Our Lady of La Leche is the patron saint of nursing mothers and women who want to become pregnant. There is a shrine in the city of St. Augustine dedicated to Mary in this role. Breastfeeding is so important, it has two patron saints, including the Blessed Mother!

Nursing in Church

Many new moms and even not so new moms feel uncomfortable breastfeeding at church and other public places. They feel torn between attending to the needs of their baby and being modest.

Nowadays, there are numerous ways to breastfeed outside the house in such a way that others have no idea what you are doing. Many home-based businesses sell stylish nursing covers. Some women wear nursing dresses or shirts that have nursing flaps and slits. Others bring a blanket or wear a sweater or shawl to help them cover up while nursing. Many moms find slings wonderful for modest nursing and for general comforting of their baby. There also the possibility of sitting in your church's library or even situating yourself next to your husband in the pew so that you are covered well.

Breastfed babies are very portable, so attending Mass requires little else besides a diaper, maybe a change of clothes for baby, and a quiet toy. Actually, comforting a baby with breastfeeding is a very non-distracting way to quiet a crying baby and is just what baby wants!

If you see a mother at Mass with a baby and one or more other children, you can offer to play quietly with her child(ren) or read to them while she nurses the baby. Another important way to help is to praise a nursing mother for her breastfeeding efforts. A positive comment can literally make someone's day! You can also bring a drink of water to a nursing mother. New mothers always appreciate meals so why not bring a meal to a mom who attends your church? One more possibility is to ask your parish priest if you can set out breastfeeding brochures in the back of church. Last but definitely not least (probably best!) is to start a nursing mothers group in your parish.

Spirituality for Busy Moms

God calls everyone to a life of prayer and holiness, not just priests and members of religious orders. The idea of including daily prayer into the busy life of motherhood can seem overwhelming. However, mothers are some of the people who most need daily, if not hourly, graces, strength and inspiration from the Holy Spirit. How can you, as a mother, then have a spiritual life while changing diapers and singing lullabies?

When is a good time to pray? If you are a morning person, how about praying before your children awake? You can pray while showering. You can pray while nursing your baby to sleep for the night or for a nap. Also, time with your child(ren) can be a prayer that doesn't

70

require a special time of day. By thinking of what Jesus would do in a situation and by trying to do just that, you are keeping Christ the center of your life.

Invocations are particularly great prayers for mothers, because they are short and can be prayed on the spot. When your child scrapes his knee, you can pray something like "Jesus, help him feel better." Or when your kids are not getting along and you are feeling overwhelmed, you can pray "Jesus, help me know what to do!" Other situations where invocations seem like just the right prayer for the moment include when an ambulance drives by, when driving past a church, and when starting a road trip.

One decade rosaries are another good fit for busy moms. Choose a decade upon which to meditate and pray it while nursing your baby or driving in the car. Fr. Sauppee wrote special rosary mysteries - the Madonna Rosary – contemplating the pregnancy, birth and nursing of Jesus. They can be found later in this chapter. Also, CNML provides one decade mothers' rosaries for those who want them for themselves or for their nursing mothers group in their parish.

The Holy Family Institute is a wonderful way for you and your spouse to grow closer to God from within your own home and to receive monthly spiritual direction from Fr. Tom Fogarty. It is a Pauline institute of secular consecrated life for married couples and for those who are widowed. One of the main focuses of the Holy Family Institute is social communication – or use of the media to spread the Gospel. Members share in the prayers of the whole Pauline family and learn how to integrate the spirituality of St. Paul; Blessed James Alberione; the Holy Family; Mary, Queen of the Apostles, and the Visit (Eucharistic adoration) into their lives. The requirements of vowed membership are minimal and are not more than a faithful Catholic already does. Plus, the annual retreat welcomes babies and children of all ages! Nursing mothers are especially plentiful! For more information, go to www.vocations-holyfamily.com

A short meditation is another valuable asset to your daily prayer time. Choose a short reading from the Bible or other book, reflect, and then talk to God about what it means to you and to your life. The next section of this book contains several Scripture verses upon which to meditate and apply to your life.

Reading the daily Scripture readings of the day - maybe with breakfast - is a great way to take part in the daily prayer of the Church even if you do not attend daily Mass.

A good way to bring closure to your day is to make an examination of conscience. This can be as short or as long as you need to make it. You can use the Ten Commandments or the seven deadly sins as a guide. Do not forget to reflect upon all the good you did during the day, too. Also, think of all the blessings God gave you during the day and say "thanks!"

Scriptural Meditations

-1-

"In her bitterness she prayed to the Lord, weeping freely, and made this vow: 'O Lord of hosts, if you look with pity on the hardship of your servant, if you remember me and do not forget me, if you give your handmaid a male child, I will give him to the Lord all the days of his life. No razor shall ever touch his head.'... She conceived and, at the end of her pregnancy, bore a son whom she named Samuel.*

"Because I asked the Lord for him. '"(1 Samuel 1:10-11, 20)

Hannah prayed for many years to conceive a baby. At that time, those who had no children were looked down upon. Hannah was so happy to give birth to and nurse a son that she dedicated Samuel to the Lord after he was weaned.

Some thoughts for meditation and living out your faith:

(1) How can I better support those couples in my parish and town who are unable to conceive? Can I pray for them? Offer an hour of adoration or a Mass?

(2) Take some time to really appreciate and enjoy your child today and the gift of breastfeeding. During your next nursing session, be truly present and savor the experience. Say a prayer of thanksgiving to Jesus for him/her.

(3) When you are tired from nursing your child yet again, remember that you are doing God's work. Just as Hannah nursed Samuel as part of his preparation for dedication to the Lord, you are doing the same.

-2-

"Blessed is the womb that bore you, and the breasts that you sucked!" (Luke 11:27)

Just as Mary was given the gift of breastfeeding the Son of God, you are breastfeeding a future saint. God gave you the privilege of leading a soul to Him. Breastfeeding nourishes your child nutritionally, emotionally and even spiritually. Through the act of breastfeeding, you show God's love to your baby and you follow God's beautiful design for motherhood.

Some ideas for living out your faith:

(1) A nursing session is a great time to pray a rosary, read Scripture or just sit in Jesus' sweet presence. Try this the next time you nurse your baby. If you have older children, naptime or bedtime nursing might be a quiet time to pray. Even just offering up your nursing time is a way to pray.

(2) Visit the Catholic Nursing Mothers League website which offers emotional and spiritual encouragement and resources for Catholic nursing mothers: www.catholicbreastfeeding.org

-3-

"...like a child quieted at its mother's breast" (Psalm 131:2)

This verse talks about quieting a baby at the breast. The breast really is a cure-all for however long the mother and child end up nursing. When the baby is very young, he wants nourishment and also to suck. As the child grows and starts to sit up, crawl and walk, he is bound to have falls. Breastfeeding is a wonderful way to take the pain away and make his world right again. Even an older child finds comfort in nursing - maybe when he is in strange surroundings or sick with the stomach flu and cannot keep anything else down.

Some thoughts for meditation and living out your faith:

(1) Think about how the Blessed Virgin Mary probably quieted baby Jesus at the breast. Although she could not really take Jesus' pain away at the crucifixion, she was able to soothe Him when He was a young child. Hopefully she found solace in that. We also may not be able to take away the hurt when our child is older and is experiencing times of unhappiness in life, but we do have the privilege of quieting him at the breast now.

(2) Send a note or card of cheer to someone you know that is experiencing illness or some sort of sadness right now.

-4-

"Going into the house they saw the child with Mary his mother, and they fell down and worshiped him" (Matthew 2:11)

Mary, Joseph, and Jesus shared a special closeness with each other. Research has shown that those first few years of life lay the foundation for the child's worldview and even their relationship with their parents. Breastfeeding can definitely help with that and it also encourages the mom and baby to stay in close proximity to each other. All those times of nursing are continually being added to your baby's emotional tank. Is it time for another deposit?

An idea for living out your faith:

(1)Visit a new mother or possibly a nursing home resident that may be feeling lonely and isolated. Bring your baby along. Everyone loves a cooing, smiley baby!

"Do not bother me; the door is now shut, and my children are with me in bed." (Luke 11:7)

Many mothers find co-sleeping a great way to breastfeed and tend to a baby or young child during the night or a nap. People from long ago and today continue this practice. Co-sleeping and nap nursing are both valuable parts of the practice of ecological breastfeeding.

Some ideas for living out your faith:

(1) If you have never considered co-sleeping and are interested in learning more, go to www.catholicbreastfeeding.org. There are several internet sites and books listed that provide scientific research and support for co-sleeping.

(2) Offer to watch a friend's baby while he sleeps so she can take a shower, go for a short walk or just take a minute for herself.

"...that you may suck and be satisfied with her consoling breasts" (Isaiah 66:11)

Notice how breastfeeding is a representative of how God consoles His children. Even in Old Testament times, breastfeeding was considered a holy activity. How much God loves babies to provide such a wonderful way to mother them. And how much God loves you too! I understand how difficult mothering can be at times, but

God is there for you - as it says in the "Footprints" poem - to carry you when you cannot go on anymore.

An idea for living out your faith:

(1)Allow another mother or your own mother to console you. Try not to think about it as burdening her but as a way she can practice the spiritual acts of mercy for Jesus.

-7-

"Can a woman forget her suckling child, that she should have no compassion on the son of her womb?" (Isaiah 49:15)

According to Scripture, God knew us in our mother's womb. As the beautiful hymn says, "Even if a mother forgets her child, He will never abandon you." Breastfeeding and encouraging other women in breastfeeding and mothering is a pro-life ministry. Not only do pregnant women need love and support, but also breastfeeding women. Let us be the face of Jesus to other pregnant and breastfeeding women, so they will truly see that God will never abandon them.

Ideas for living out your faith:

(1) Abortion is such a tragedy in today's society. Donate money to a pro-life cause, donate baby items to your local crisis pregnancy center, or sign an online pro-life petition sometime this week.

(2) Call or visit a single mother you know.

"although we were able to impose our weight as apostles of Christ. Rather, we were gentle among you, as a nursing mother cares for her children."(1 Thes 2:7)

During breastfeeding, hormones are released in the mother's body that help her to relax and sometimes even want to fall asleep! I believe that breastfeeding helps mothers to be gentler with their child. How easy it is for parents to get frustrated - I know I have felt that way many times over the years. However, sitting down to nurse a baby or a toddler seems to make life feel just a little bit better. I can often handle the next crisis in a gentler manner and behave more similarly to how St. Paul treated his fellow Christians.

Ideas for living your faith:

(1) Memorize the Scripture verse. When the next crisis or frustrating moment occurs, try to remember St. Paul's words and handle the situation in a gentler manner than you may feel like reacting.

(2) If you see a mother in public looking embarrassed by her toddler's tantrum, go up to her and tell her you know how she feels. Let her know that your toddler has done that many times, too. Maybe even ask her if there is anything you can do to help her through it. She will remember your kindness for the rest of the day and afterwards!

9

"She leaned over close to him and, in derision of the cruel tyrant, said in their native language: "Son, have pity on me, who carried you in my womb for nine months, nursed you for three years, brought you up, educated and supported you to your present age." (2 Maccabees 7:27)

This verse shows how extended breastfeeding was the norm in the Old Testament times. It really is today's Western world that frowns upon this practice. It is interesting how acceptable or unacceptable different activities are depending on the time period and country in which you live. However, there are certain things written in our hearts - like our faith in Jesus Christ - and as part of our nature – breastfeeding and the preciousness of human life - that we should let no society devalue. If you are nursing a baby or toddler right now, remember that you are following God's special plan!

Ideas for living your faith:

(1) Remind the mother of a nursing toddler how wonderful it is she is responding to her child's continued need to nurse.

(2) Start a nursing mothers group in your parish and discuss the benefits of extended breastfeeding at a meeting. CNML provides an online guide that makes leading meetings easy.

Father Sauppe's Theotokos Chaplet
(Imprimatur: Most Reverend Daniel R. Jenky, 2 February 2006)

Using ordinary rosary beads…

Pray this version of the "Hail Mary" on the small beads:

Hail Mary,
Full of grace,
The Lord is with thee;
Blessed art thou among women, and
Blessed is the fruit of thy womb, Jesus.
Holy Mary,
Mother of God (Theotokos),
Blessed is the womb that carried Jesus
And the breasts that nursed him.
Blessed are those who hear
The word of God and keep it.

The Five Mysteries of the Maternity of Mary:

The Quickening: the Blessed Mother feels Jesus' first movements in the womb

His First Nursing: the Blessed Mother gives her infant His first nourishment

His First Steps: Jesus takes his first steps towards His destiny – His passion and cross

His First Words: Jesus speaks His first words

Jesus is Weaned: the last breast-fed bond between Mother and Son

Lenten Fasting Guidelines
for Breastfeeding Moms

According to several good Catholic websites, including EWTN, women who are currently breastfeeding are not required to take part in the usual fast from food on Ash Wednesday and Good Friday. In the place of fasting from food, you can still take part in the "spirit of the rule" by giving up something else such as internet use, TV watching, buying unnecessary items, etc. Actually, if you are concerned with the media's influence on society and like the idea of fasting from it during Lent, you might be a good candidate for membership in the Holy Family Institute as previously discussed. Another possibility is to donate the monetary value of the meals you eat on Ash Wednesday and Good Friday to the poor. This would share in the "almsgiving" aspect of Lent. Lastly, you might also consider praying more, which can easily be done while nursing a baby and is another important part of our Lenten journey. The Madonna rosary decade or the meditations listed earlier in this book are good starting places. Nursing mothers can have a holy Lent even when not fasting!

Chapter 5: Mothers' Stories

Sunday

by Marian Tascio Friedrichs,
mother to Isaiah, Bernadette, Kateri and baby on the
way

He starts asking as soon as we reach our pew. "Mama, wanna do nook. Wanna do noook."

I glance at the nearest faces. They're all bent over hymnals or turned toward the aisle, where Father sings with gusto behind the blank-faced, decidedly non-singing altar servers. I check the Baby Girl beside us. She is perched in her father's arms, nibbling with hearty interest a button on his red-checked shirt. It is the same shirt he wore on our first date, when we smiled nervously at one another over roast chicken and sweet potato fries.

"Mama, do nook. Do nook, nook, nook, nooook!" The Little Boy is tugging on my shirt now, his upturned face a study in urgency.

"OK," I whisper. "Just as soon as everyone sits down." I scoop him up so he can see what's going on. He sucks on my collar and gazes absently at the doings up front: the kissing of the altar, the settling of the people into their places. He whimpers his request a few more times during the opening prayers, and I promise soon, soon.

At last we sit, and he nestles into my lap. He is still a baby, this Little Boy who became a big brother one morning and turned two years old thirteen days later. At his birthday party he fell asleep in my lap, just like this, as the cake was being served. We have a picture of his father offering the cake to his curled-up figure. There are colored sprinkles and two candles, and beneath the white frosting, there is chocolate. But at that moment he needed only Mama. And Mama means this.

I lift my shirt, keeping my head down and hoping everyone around us is as rapt by the scripture readings as my Baby Girl is by the lights in the high ceiling. He snuggles in and latches. I listen to the readings, too.

We make it halfway through the homily before my Little Boy's sister notices what he is doing and begins some whimpering of her own. Daddy and I trade off; the Baby Girl leans into me while the Little Boy sits beside his father, flips through a baby Bible and munches Cheerios, his face flushed with contentment. Filled, he has yielded to his sister without complaint.

I am grateful for that. Nursing them both at once is something I only do in certain places; it requires a lot of space, a lot of exposure, and only understanding witnesses. Typically, when we "do nook all together", the Little Boy and Baby Girl have ignored each other, but sometimes these days she toys with his hair and he laughs. Lately they have been finding each other's fingertips, exploring nails and knuckles, holding hands briefly as they top off their tanks of mother-love side by side.

The moment is coming. Daddy kneels; Little Boy stands on the kneeler and rests his chin on the back of the pew in front of us; I bow my head. Baby Girl feels so light in my arms after her big brother, but now her body grows heavy with encroaching sleep.

"Take this, all of you, and eat it. This is my body, which will be given up for you."

I touch my heart; the Baby Girl begins her deep gulping. I ache a little as the milk lets down, and I think about my bones. I read somewhere that they break down a bit when we start feeding our first babies, but then the bones are replenished and become stronger than before. I picture the cells—white and spongy—drifting apart, giving themselves to the outflow that will become my children's food and drink, only to regroup and regain one another—finding life by losing it.

"Take this, all of you, and drink from it. This is the cup of my blood, the blood of the new and everlasting covenant, which will be shed for you and for all…"

She has stopped gulping. A droplet of milk escapes her slackening mouth. My blood. That's what it's made from. My life becomes her life. Her eyelids flutter slightly but stay closed. She hasn't let go of my breast. It will be a trick, carrying her to the altar while keeping her asleep and myself covered up, but I've done it before many times.

I stand when our turn comes and whisper my usual prayer: "Take away my heart of stone and replace it with a heart of flesh." I am begging to become what I eat.

And afterwards, while He melts inside me: "Body of Christ, save me. Blood of Christ, inebriate me…"

Later, as we file out the doors, Little Boy asks for another turn. The day is nearly half gone, and he is eager for rest and reconnection. But we tell him where we are going next, and thoughts of mama-milk give way to the anticipation of Grandma's house, where there will be aunts and uncles, lunch and cake for Daddy's birthday.

Twenty minutes into the drive, Baby Girl wakes up in her car seat. No one is touching her. No one is holding her. She does not know where we are. She begins to cry.

Her brother says, "She needs nook."

He's STILL Nursing?

by Maureen Armendariz,
mother to Isaiah, Rosie, John Paul and Ivy

When a toddler nurses...

I feel my cheeks going red....Over the shouts and shrieks of children playing on the equipment, I catch broken bits of the conversation at another table.

"...nursing that kid?" "(Gasp) Yes! I can't believe people do that!" "And in public..."

And I purposely shut my ears.

I drop my head and sniff the blonde head pressed up against me.

Smells like heaven and earth combined.

A moment ago he was a wild toddler, sweaty from his antics, unsure of what he wanted from me, sure of everything he didn't want (anything and everything). But finally he slowed down. And before I knew it, he was clinging to my leg whimpering, "Paaa, eee," (our strange code-word for nurse, please.) So we left the big kids playing on the jungle gym and found a bench for a nurse-rest.

It's really impossible to explain to a woman who hasn't done it herself- why would you want to nurse a big, cranky toddler? Oh, sure, they get demanding. Oh, sure, it's inconvenient at times. Oh, sure, sometimes you'd love to sleep curled up in a ball instead of tangled up with a kicking little body.

But.

But it's the love pats on the arm while he suckles.

But it's the change from meltdown to smiles after a tumble when he only latches on for half a minute. But it's talking with a friend while you effortlessly nurse him to sleep. But it's the eyes that gaze up at you adoringly- looking at you the same way he has thousands of times over the last two years.

I think of all the things a mom misses when she and her baby wean at 6 months, or 12 months. All the special, secret things that pass between a mother and her child during those silent moments. (As a friend of mine jokes, "It's the only time she holds still!") And I'm not embarrassed anymore. Instead I feel a compassionate longing that every mother might know the peace and joy of nursing a toddler. And I lift my head up from my son's, look across the grass, and smile brightly at the moms sitting over there.

The Benefits of the Seven Standards of Ecological Breastfeeding

by Judith Dunne, mother to Joy

The first positive experience of using one of the Seven Standards of Ecological Breastfeeding, namely co-sleeping, was when my baby was a couple of weeks old. I am most definitely NOT a night owl and would normally be in bed or asleep by 10 pm and sleep right through until 6:30/7 AM. The way it had been recommended in a lot of books of having your baby in a cot /crib/moses basket nearby, didn't work very well for me as I would be sheer exhausted getting up to nurse her. When I learned how to breastfeed AND sleep with my baby, it was a sheer joy and my husband was soon on board when he realized the positives of it all- little night disturbance and waking to see his beautiful baby beside him.

Another positive of the Seven Standards of ecological breastfeeding is the bonding aspect of unrestricted nursing. It makes me stop and relax for a bit and just enjoy my baby. If I was bottle feeding or using pacifiers, I am sure she and I would miss out on learning more about our little nuances and daily growth emotionally, physically and spiritually. I would probably rush around "doing " all the time rather than making the time for just "being" with my baby.

It is also a very humbling experience to actually have to put aside for a little while your own goals for the day, when you know your baby needs you more. It helps me grow in virtue and God always knows how much I can handle in any given day.

Ecological Breastfeeding: Its Value for Childhood Leukemia

by Pam Pilch, founder of the Catholic Nursing Mothers League

I discovered ecological breastfeeding from reading Sheila Kippley's book, *Breastfeeding and Natural Child*

Spacing, while still pregnant with my first child. At the time I had no idea how much the information and lifestyle and practices would come to mean to me. With my first son, I put the Seven Standards of Ecological Breastfeeding into practice. We enjoyed a happy, healthy breastfeeding relationship and realized all the many benefits, included extended natural breastfeeding infertility. My first son nursed for nearly 3 years – until he weaned on his own during my second pregnancy.

As the years passed, my second son came along, nursed for 3 years, until HIS baby brother, Jonathan, was born. We enjoyed the closeness, the warmth, the attachment – not to mention the health benefits. All went well and by the time our third baby was born, we were pretty much in a rhythm.

My third son, Jonathan, nursed easily right away, just as his brothers had. But something we never expected happened to him when we was just 2-and-a-half years old. He was diagnosed, at that young age, with leukemia.

The leukemia diagnosis was a huge (and awful) surprise to our family. Up until that time, Jonathan (a champion nurser like his brothers before him) had been perfectly happy and healthy. He had never had so much as an ear infection, never been hospitalized (not even for his birth – his was a normal and healthy homebirth!), never taken an antibiotic, not even once. It seemed to creep up quietly – over the course of a few weeks, he seemed tired, just a little under-the-weather. He didn't want to run around so much, wouldn't climb up his play structure, wanted to be carried up and down the stairs. But there was no dramatic change in his health. We were sure it was only a virus – a "bug" going around. Finally though, after a week or so, I decided to call the pediatrician "just in case." As soon as we arrived, the doctor performed some blood work and told us that Jonathan was very seriously ill, and we would need to be transported immediately from her office by ambulance to the main teaching hospital in our region. I asked if Jonathan was going to be okay, and she replied, "I don't know."

Terrified, we climbed into the ambulance. And while the EMTs were starting Jonathan's IV, he asked to nurse. I looked at the EMT to see if it was okay, and he said, "My wife is still nursing our 9-month-old, and no telling when she'll quit! Please - do nurse him. It will be the best thing for both of you." We nursed in the ambulance, then in the Emergency Room, then through the ordeal of being told by the doctor that our baby had leukemia.

We nursed day and night, in the hospital (where I was blessed to be able to stay 24 hours a day due to the support of family and friends who stepped in to care for my older children full-time) where his condition was stabilized and his chemotherapy started. Except for when he needed to fast in preparation for a surgical procedure, Jonathan nursed frequently, almost like a newborn again. My milk supply, which had been waning, began to rebound. As the medications and the process of his body eliminating the dead leukemia cells made him feel sicker and sicker, nursing became his main comfort - and mine too.

In the first days of having a child diagnosed with cancer, the worst feeling I think for a mother is one of helplessness. You feel that this thing has attacked your child, and that there is NOT ONE THING you can do about it. But the good thing about breastfeeding is that you ARE doing something. Even if your child is very, very sick, you are providing him with the stability and comfort that he has known all his life, even in the midst of great upheaval and pain and fear. You are giving him some (even if only a very little bit of) nutrition and fluid, and plenty of closeness and comfort – not to mention all the good hormones you stimulate to make him (and you!) feel calm in the midst of the storm. In one of the worst and scariest moments of mothering, nursing my critically-ill toddler turned out to be the one thing I COULD do for him. And I thanked God for this blessing.

After his initial intensive treatment, Jonathan's continued treatment suppressed his immune system and made him vulnerable to infection. After he came home, we continued to nurse, still day and night. And his oncologist commended me, telling me that the antibodies my milk was able to pass to him were probably really helping him avoid fevers and infections common to leukemia patients.

Now his treatment has continued for six months, and he is through the worst. We are in a long-term maintenance phase, in which he still receives chemotherapy. His prognosis is, so far as we can tell, excellent. And in July, he turned 3, and he is still nursing. We will let Jonathan lead the way in weaning, as we have done for his brothers before. But this time, we see him nurse and we see how even in a critical time, the nursing relationship has infinite value.

I hope that no other breastfeeding mothers ever have to see their children suffer with a cancer diagnosis or any other serious illness. But I do have to say that as much as I have always appreciated the general benefits of breastfeeding, I have never appreciated them more than I have in the past six months. I'm so glad that I had the information and support to continue breastfeeding past the first year of Jonathan's life - I never knew what nursing would mean to both of us in the future.

Note: Pam's son is in remission and has had a clean bill of health for the last several years!

Feed My Sheep

by Andrea Nease,
mom of Stanlee, Isaiah and Hannah

I grew up in the south, the Bible belt. I went to a myriad of churches growing up, mostly Baptist, with some Pentecostal and non-denominational mixed it.

In my teenage years I fell very much in love...with a very devout Catholic. This wonderful man made it clear that he would never marry a non-Catholic. Lacking maturity, and having a more relativistic view on religion, I agreed to become Catholic (just to get married). I went through the RCIA classes, and was confirmed in Easter of '07. We were married that December.

Through the entire process, I never really believed much of what the Catholic Church taught, aside from the basics we had in common. My husband's reverence for the Eucharist is amazing, and this subject was commonly talked about when religion came up in conversation. There were many things I was out-right opposed to. One item in particular was infant baptism. However, the Church's teachings on the Eucharist did not bother me, although I was really indifferent about the whole thing. "So what if it's Jesus' body? It doesn't matter to me if it is or isn't. You say it is? Okay, fine," I thought.

Then we had kids, and I started to take things a little more seriously. I really wanted to do right by my kids. My husband wanted to baptize our infant son, and this bothered me. During that time, we made a compromise that our son would be baptized as an infant, but we were not going to circumcise him. My husband got what he wanted, I got what I wanted, and my son....well, baptism certainly wasn't going to hurt him, even if it wasn't "real".

Adjusting to motherhood was difficult for me. I was extremely exhausted, had never changed a diaper in my life, had no support or family close to me, and had a very unhappy baby, which I now know would be defined as "high needs." We had some problems with breastfeeding in the beginning, but because of my innate stubbornness given to me by God (and also to my first child), we stuck with it. I truly did not enjoy breastfeeding at all. I looked forward to when I could wean at the 1 year-mark. I was pressured by pediatricians to minimize my son's nursing sessions early on, and let him cry-it-out so I could actually get some sleep (which didn't work, by the way). During these times, I was always encouraged to wean whenever I expressed hardships with nursing by family and my husband alike, but we persevered.

When my son Stanlee was 8 months old, we started cosleeping because I just couldn't take being a walking zombie anymore. I nursed him back to sleep at night when he woke, which was frequently, but I still tried to limit his nursing during the day. My periods came back at this time, even though I was still nursing every 3-4 hours during the day and at least every 2 hours at night.

When Stanlee was 12 months old, I slowly started introducing goat's milk in a sippy cup to start the weaning process. My son didn't really care for that, so I started researching how to wean on the internet. On accident, I stumbled across a Christian article that talked about what the Bible had to say about weaning. I learned that the Bible referenced nursing a three year old, and this surprised me. I then started researching nursing older children, and found out that it's natural and healthier. I also started reading comments about "nursing on demand", and how women nursed their babies whenever the baby wanted, and didn't count feedings or watch the clock.

I decided to continue nursing and let my son self-wean. He was right at the age where he started to point to express his needs, and started pointing at my chest when he wanted to nurse. This was a turning point for us, because before I never really knew what his cries meant. This was a clear indication he wanted to nurse. God magically put all the pieces together, right at the same time, to help me understand.

The same day I read that article, which was the same day my son started pointing at my chest to nurse, I started nursing him on demand. He never sucked his thumb from that moment forward. He had been sucking it since he was 3 months old (around the time I started trying to stretch out his feedings). I instantly knew that I had failed him. I hadn't nursed him when he needed me - I had left him to himself to take care of his sucking needs. Of course it wasn't intentional; I was just an uneducated mother trying to figure things out by myself. Looking back, I wish I could have changed many things with my first child. But I am so grateful God gave me Stanlee first. Stanlee is exactly the baby I needed to teach me some valuable lessons. Had I been given a less intense, easier going baby the first time around, I probably would have weaned at one year or earlier, and missed out on some great lessons.

I was barely getting the hang of things when I found out I was pregnant with our second child, Isaiah, when Stanlee was 19 months old. Stanlee had just gone through a random nursing strike (during the day time) for a couple weeks. I thought he was self-weaning. Wrong. He was back to nursing 24/7 after those couple weeks. I'm not sure if my cycles before this were anovulatory or not, but I think it's possible the nursing strike caused my fertility to really return and conceive again. I had started practicing ecological breastfeeding with Stanlee from 12 months old on; it may have kept my fertility at bay until the nursing strike.

Anyway, the anticipation of a new child brought unresolved religious issues back to the surface. Would we do infant baptism again? I still wasn't comfortable, but knew it was non-negotiable for my husband. I needed answers. Not only on this issue, but others we disagreed on. We couldn't both be right. I spent several months digging deep, researching, and trying to find the right answers.

Long story short (and sparing you the details of some shouting matches between my husband and I), I recognized the authority of the Catholic Church and had a major conversion. I stopped going up to receive the Eucharist because I hadn't gone to confession (not even before I was confirmed). With 2 years of nursing under my belt at that time, I knew what a major sacrifice giving your body to another person is.

I finally "got" the Eucharist.

I don't just symbolically feed my babies at the breast. It is my actual body, in direct contact with my child's body. This gift of my body helps grow and nurture life according to God's will, not mine. In the Eucharist, I also have a real, tangible, physical relationship with Him. It took me a long time to appreciate nursing, but I finally got there. Once I stopped withholding myself from my baby, and nursed him whenever he needed, I saw how much happier he was. He cried less and started growing better physically and developmentally. His growth had slowed when I had used cry-it-out methods and restricted his nursing to a schedule. Over time, he started trusting me more. Nothing really changed, except I put myself in my son's shoes, and realized how important nursing was to him. How happy it made him. How much he needed it. How it helped him grow. Nursing was still difficult from my end and a sacrifice, but it was worth it to see him happy, and to see how it benefitted him. Now we had lots of giggling, playing, and bonding at the breast instead of a countdown for him to get off of me.

Knowing how difficult it can be to nurse a child, and how difficult it can be nursing two children as I am tandem nursing both my boys now, it blows my mind how Jesus sacrifices His own body for millions with the Eucharist. Willingly. I complain about nursing, and His sacrifice puts me to shame and keeps me humble. I'm not indifferent about receiving Holy Communion anymore. I AM NOT WORTHY.

I look forward to going to Mass, so I can be "nursed" by Jesus through the Holy Eucharist. I need Him. There are times I need to go to Confession before I can receive. Confession still terrifies me so unfortunately I tend to put it off. Whenever I am in a Eucharist "drought", everything seems to go wrong and have a horrible snowball effect. When I'm able to receive the Eucharist, I can see His grace working in my life. Helping me grow spiritually, just as nursing my children helps them grow. The Eucharist brings me a sense of peace, as nursing my children helps them calm down and feel safe and secure in my arms.

When children go through a growth spurt, they increase their nursing. When we need to increase the graces we receive, and grow more spiritually, receiving the Eucharist more frequently can help us with our "growth spurt". I would love to be able to go to daily Mass, but it has been a struggle just to keep myself going every Sunday after years of only going when it suited me.

It's really hard to put into words what the Eucharist does for you. People outside the faith struggle to understand it and question why it's so important to us Catholics. Actually, even some Catholics themselves don't understand the Eucharist well or "get it". Those of us who know are drawn to it. Crave it. We look forward to when we can get it again.

In the same way, our little children need to nurse "just because" and can't always explain to us why they need to nurse. Sometimes I get frustrated with how often my children want to nurse. I've asked my oldest several times in the past WHY he wants to nurse. Is he hungry? Is he thirsty? Is he sad? Does he miss me? Is he tired? I go on and on, but never figure out why he wants to nurse most of the time. My son can't explain it either, but nursing just brings him peace and satisfies him. Sometimes we don't even know consciously we need it, but once we receive it, things have changed. Nursing can make a screaming toddler turn into a sweet, giggly, happy child. Mom too, for that matter! Sometimes our children are so upset and overwhelmed with their emotions, it is simply a job too big for them to handle on their own. In these times, our nurslings look to Mom to be there to help them. After I've thought about my sins, and how I need to be more holy, and I'm walking up for communion, all that is going through my head is "I can't do this by myself, Lord. I need Your help. I need You. Help me!" Jesus is there for us, and comforts us, just as a nursing mother comforts her child.

I often see young mothers my age, who do not nurse their children, really struggle with dealing with their little ones. Now, parenting is never easy for parents, and some children are more difficult than others. Nursing mothers do not have perfect children by any means, nor are they perfect parents. However, nursing mothers have a wonderful blessing and an extra tool in their toolbox they can use to parent their children through the nursing relationship. Before I nursed my oldest on demand, he was always upset and I was constantly trying to do things or find objects that would make him happy all day long. Car rides, walking, rocking, singing to him, toys, strollers, food, snacks, drinks, cuddling, reading, etc, etc. Nothing really helped him until I started meeting his nursing needs. Of course there are children who are easier to pacify than others, but still there is something special about nursing that sets it apart from any other "trick", that provides something special none of those other things can. I've witnessed when children have lost their pacifiers and become hysterical and the mother is unable to console her child. I'm so glad I cannot misplace my breasts. Now that my oldest is almost 4 years old, I can't imagine getting through the toddler years and tantrums without having the option to nurse! In a similar way, if I did not go to a Catholic Church, and was not able to receive Communion, no matter what church I went to, it would not be able to give me the comfort the Eucharist can provide. I still may hear a good sermon and have good fellowship, but it is lacking and incomplete.

During Mass tonight, I tried to think of some more similarities between nursing and the Eucharist. We usually sit in the back, so it can be a slow walk up to the front, which seems to last forever. It reminded me of how nursing babies have to work a little harder to make our milk let down, instead of it flowing freely from a bottle. Even if you sit up front and don't have a long wait in line, we still have to work and do our part by making sure we are worthy to receive and go to Confession if needed beforehand, which can be a lot of work, and showing up to Mass. We have to cooperate with God and do our part.

Once I get to the priest, I focus all my attention on the Body of Christ, and feel relief and peace as soon as I receive the Body. This reminds me of my nurslings too. My boys can be quite active and distracted at the breast at times, but they are always focused on me the moment my milk lets down and they start swallowing, even if they start wiggling and playing after the let-down has subsided. They usually look up at me, into my eyes. This reminds me of when the priest is consecrating the Body and Blood and raising it up for His children to see. At that moment, we look up to Jesus, the Shepherd feeding His sheep. Jesus and His bride (the Church) feed us, the lost sheep. But nursing mothers everywhere feed His sheep, too, in the home- the domestic church. They prepare His children to receive God's message by providing trust and love which helps them grow in Christ.

Most mothers reading this will know the natural age of weaning is 2-7 years. In reality they never really wean, as usually soon after they wean from the breast they reach the age of reason and commonly partake in their first Communion. In Hebrews 5:12-14 we read about how it's necessary for us to learn the basics (the milk) before we can learn the meatier truths of the faith (the solid food). Mothers everywhere have an incredibly important job in nursing their babies and building a solid foundation so their children (God's children) can grow, be holy, and be part of the Body of Christ. Nursing mothers are reminded during the Eucharist that their hard work and sacrifice they make are not in vain.

Now, I understand and listen when my husband excitedly talks about the Eucharist, and he better understands why nursing is so important now that we can see the similarities between the two. I am happy to report my husband no longer recommends me to wean when the going gets tough with nursing. He also says I never have to worry about someone saying something to me if I'm nursing in public because he will "take care of it". I also half-joke with him that he is under strict orders to practice male lactation in the event of my death. Strangely, he doesn't confidently say he'll take care of that one!

Chapter 6: About the Catholic Nursing Mothers League (CNML)

CNML was founded in April 2006 by Pamela Pilch, who was inspired by Sheila Kippley's work concerning ecological breastfeeding. Sheila suggested in her book, *Breastfeeding and Catholic Motherhood*, that someone with a passion for breastfeeding could start a nursing mothers group in her parish. Soon after the release of that book, Pam began laying the groundwork for such an organization.

Pamela Pilch's plan for CNML was to provide encouragement and resources for Catholic mothers to gather in parishes, to learn about breastfeeding and mothering, to give and receive emotional and spiritual support, and to reach out to parishes and communities to educate about the many physical and relational benefits, and about the long-standing Church teaching in support of maternal breastfeeding.

Pam authored the CNML principles, faith statement, mission and goals. She arranged for its first website, its legal classification as a non-profit organization in the state of Michigan, the CNMLchat Yahoo group, the board of directors, and the advisory board, of which I was a part nearly from the beginning.

After prayer and consideration, Pam decided to hand off the running of CNML to me; this took place over the summer of 2009. Since I took over as Executive Director of CNML, the ministry has slowly grown. It now has a new and improved website, a blog, a Facebook group and page, an online Resource Guide for Starting a Catholic

Mothers Group, and legal classification as a 501(c)(3) in the state of New Mexico.

Would you like to encourage breastfeeding women and to help them grow into the beautiful mothers God is calling them to become? Do you feel called to start a nursing mothers group in your parish? It really does not take much time at all. There are resources on the CNML website that make it very easy to implement. You can also use this book to help answer basic breastfeeding or ecological breastfeeding questions. All you need to do is ask for God's guidance and show up for an hour or two once per month! If you need freebies such as copies of Sheila Kippley's three breastfeeding books, Our Lady of La Leche medals and holy cards, or one decade rosaries, please contact CNML.

Principles of the
Catholic Nursing Mothers League

God the Creator has a plan for all men, women and children and this plan applies to every area of our lives. The Catholic Church's authoritative teaching helps us to know this plan. God's plan includes conception, childbirth and the nurturing of babies.

Breastfeeding is the natural continuation of the childbearing cycle which begins with conception, pregnancy and childbirth. As such, it forms an important part of God's plan for mothers and babies.

Breast milk is the best nourishment for babies and the act of breastfeeding provides the best nurturing environment for both mothers and babies.

Breastfeeding is a special way in which a mother makes a sincere gift of herself to her baby. Breastfeeding is also a special way in which mothers are called to serve life in one of its most vulnerable stages. In the breastfeeding Madonna, Catholic mothers have a special exemplar. Ecological breastfeeding - the form of mothering which tends to delay the return of fertility after the birth of a baby - benefits the nursing child, and enhances the mother's health and well-being. Its natural child spacing effect is a moral and healthy form of natural birth regulation and should be supported and encouraged by families, society and the Church.

Children deserve to be raised to appreciate the equality and complementarity of men and women in the context of life-long marriage. Fathers offer essential spiritual and emotional support to their breastfeeding wives, and they provide for and protect the nursing couple. These early acts of service lay the groundwork for fathers' unique and irreplaceable role in their children's lives.

Women have a right to be truthfully informed about the benefits of breastfeeding for themselves as well as for their babies. Families, parishes, communities, governments and society have a responsibility to protect and strengthen cultural support for breastfeeding practices.

Children need their mothers' presence, especially in the first three years of life. With or without breastfeeding, motherhood is an important and valuable way in which women live in accordance with their nature as persons created in God's image.

Faith Statement of the
Catholic Nursing Mothers League

The Catholic Nursing Mothers League acknowledges that the Catholic Church was founded by Christ, and the League assents to all that
the Church authentically teaches through the Magisterium.

The teachings of the Roman Pontiffs and the Congregation for the Doctrine of the Faith are accepted by CNML as authoritative.

In particular, the Catholic Nursing Mothers League assents to the following specific teachings that bear on our work as supporters of breastfeeding
mothers:

1. We respect the sanctity of all human life from conception to natural death. We oppose all forms of abortion, both surgical and via abortifacient devices and drugs.
2. We believe that marriage is between one man and one woman and that children are the supreme gift of marriage. We believe that married couples are called to be generous in the service of life and to exercise responsible parenthood.
3. We reject all unnatural forms of birth control, and we reject as contrary to God's plan all means of seeking conception in which technological interventions are substituted for the marriage act. We accept the morality of natural means of birth regulation for couples with a serious reason to space their children.

References

Kippley, Sheila. *Breastfeeding and Catholic Motherhood.* Manchester: Sophia Institute Press, 2005. Print.

Kippley, Sheila. *The Seven Standards of Ecological Breastfeeding: The Frequency Factor.* lulu.com, 2008. Print.

Sears, Dr. William, Martha, Dr. Robert, Dr. James. *The Baby Book, Revised and Updated Edition: Everything You Need to Know About Your Baby from Birth to Age Two.* Little, Brown and Company, *2013.* Print.

The Holy Bible, Revised Standard Version, Catholic Edition, Thomas Nelson Publishers for Ignatius Press, 1966. (Scriptural meditations 2-7)

New American Bible Revised Edition. Saint Benedict Press. Web. 2011. (Scriptural meditations 1, 8 and 9)

A Few Scientific Studies

dental problems

Leite-Cavalcanti, A. et al. 2007. Breastfeeding, bottle-feeding, sucking habits and malocclusion in Brazilian preschool children. *Rev Salud Publica 9(2):194-204.*

vision problems

Agostini, C. and M. Giovannini. 2001. Cognitive and visual development: influence of differences in breast and formula fed infants. *Nutr Health* 15(3-4):183.

allergies

Muche-Borowski, C. et al. 2009. Allergy prevention. *J Dtsch Dermatolog Ges* 106(39):625-631.

Crohn's disease and ulcerative colitis

Barclay, A.R. 2009. Systematic review: the role of breastfeeding in the development of pediatric inflammatory bowel disease. *J Pediatr* 155(3):421-426.

leukemia

Bener, A. et al. 2008. Does prolonger breastfeeding reduce the risk for childhood leukemia and lymphomas? *Minerva Pediatr* 60(2):155-161.

type 1 diabetes

Vaiva S. et al. 2004. Longer breastfeeding is an independent protective factor against development of type 1 diabetes mellitus in childhood. *Diabetes/Metabolism Research and Reviews* 20(2):150-157.

type 2 diabetes

Pettit, D.J. et al. 1997. Breastfeeding and the incidence of non-insulin dependent diabetes mellitus in Pima Indians. *Lancet* 350:166-168.

ear infections

Sabirov, A. et al. 2009. Breastfeeding is associated with a reduced frequency of acute otitis media and high serum antibody levels against NTHi and outer membrane protein vaccine antigen candidate P6. *Pediatr Res* 66(5):565.

severe diarrhea and necrotizing enterocolitis

Dujits, L. et al. 2009. Breastfeeding protects against infectious diseases during infancy in industrialized countries. A systematic review. *Matern Child Nutr* 5(3):199-210.

obesity

O'Tierney, P.F. et al. 2009. Duration of breastfeeding and adiposity in adult life. *J Nutr* 139(2):422S-425S.

SIDS

Venemann, M.M. et al. 2009. Does breastfeeding reduce the risk of sudden infant death syndrome? *Pediatrics* 123(3):e406-e410.

osteoporosis (child)

Jones, G. et al. 2000. Breastfeeding in early life and bone mass in prepubertal children: a longitudinal study. *Osteoporosis Int* 11(2):146-152.

IQ

Kramer, M.S. 2008. Breastfeeding and child cognitive development: new evidence from a large randomized trial. *Arch Gen Psychiatry* 65(5):578-584.

heart disease

Parikh, N.H. et al. 2009. Breastfeeding in fancy and adult cardiovascular disease risk factors. *Am J Med* 122(7):656-663.

living cells in breast milk

Goldman, A.S. et al. 1990. Anti-inflammatory systems in human milk. *Adv Exp Med Biol 262:69-76.*

breast cancer

Collaborative Group on Hormonal Factors in Breast Cancer. 2002. Breast cancer and breastfeeding:

collaborative reanalysis of individual date from 47 epidemiological studies in 30 countires, including 50,302 women with breast cancer and 96,973 women without the disease. *Lancet 360(9328):187-195.*

ovarian cancer

Danforth, K.N. et al. 2007. Breastfeeding and risk of ovarian cancer in two prospective cohorts. *Cancer Causes Control* 18(5):517-523.

rheumatoid arthritis

Pikwer, M. et al. 2009. Breastfeeding, but not use of oral contraceptives, is associated with a reduced risk of rheumatoid arthritis. *Ann Rheum Dis* 68(4):526-530.

metabolic syndrome

Stuebe, A.M. and J.W. Rich-Edwards. 2009. The reset hypothesis: lactation and maternal metabolism. *Am J Perinatol* 26(1)81-88.

insulin-dependent diabetic mothers likely to need less insulin while nursing

Riviello, C. et al. 2009. Breastfeeding and the basal insulin requirement in type 1 diabetic women. *Endocr Pract* 15(3):187-193.

high blood pressure

Jonas, W. et al. 2008. Short- and long-term decrease of blood pressure in women during breastfeeding. *Breastfeeding Med* 3(2):103-109.

osteoporosis and fractures (mother)

Lopez, J. M. et al. 1996. Bone turnover and density in healthy women during breastfeeding and after weaning. *Osteoporos Int* 6:153-159.

inverted nipples

Patel, Y. 2008. Inverted nipples: correction using a simple disposable syringe. *East Afr Med J* 85(1):51-52.

doulas

Hodnett, E.D. et al. 2007. Continuous support for women during childbirth. *Cochrane Database Syst Rev* 18(3):CD003766.

excess IV fluids and breast engorgement

Academy of Breastfeeding Medicine Protocol Committee. Berens, P. 2009. ABM clinical protocol #20: Engorgement. *Breastfeeding Med* 4(2):111-113.

frequency of breastfeedings

Kent, J. et al. 2006. Volume and frequency of breastfeedings and fat content of breast milk throughout the day. *Pediatrics* 117(3):e387-e395.

number of wet diapers and bowel movements

Nommsen-Rivers, L.A. et al. 2008. Newborn wet and soiled diaper counts and timing of onset of lactation as indicators of breastfeeding adequacy. *J Hum Lact* 24(1):27-33.

normal weight gain

Crossland, D.S. et al. 2008. Weight change in the term baby in the first 2 weeks of life. *Acta Paediatr 97(4):425-429.*

baby's weight loss after birth

Martens, P.J. and Romphf. 2007. Factors associated with newborn in-hospital weight loss:comparisons by feeding methods, demographics, and birthing procedures. *J Hum Lact* 23(3):233-241.

maternal fluid intake while nursing

Dusdieker, L. et al. 1985. Effect of supplemental fluids on human milk production. *J Pediatr* 106(2):207-211.

taste of milk after exercise

Wallace, J.P. et al. 2009. Infant acceptance of postexercise breast milk. *Pediatrics* 89(6 Pt 2):1245-1247.

alcohol

Koren, G. 2002. Drinking alcohol while breastfeeding: will it harm my baby? *Canadian Family Physician* 48:39-41.

orthodontia

Page, D.C. 2001. Breastfeeding in early functional jaw orthopedics. *Funct Orthod* 18(3):24-27.

lactational amenorrhea method (LAM)

Perez, A, Labbok, M.,Queenan, J. 1992. Clinical Study of the lactational amenorrhoea method for family planning. *The Lancet* 339(8799):968-970.

effect of pacifier use on the return of fertility

Ingram, J. et al. 2004. The association of progesterone, infant formula use and pacifier use with the return of menstruation in breastfeeding women. *European Journal of Obsetrics& Gynecology and Reproductive Biology* 114(2):197-202.

effect of suckling on lactational amenorrhea

Taylor, William et al. 1999. Continuously recorded suckling behavior and its Effect on Lactational Amenorrhoea. *Journal of Biosocial Science* 31:289-310.

cosleeping, SIDS and breastfeeding

Mckenna, J. et al. 2007. Mother-Infant Cosleeping, Breastfeeding and Sudden Infant Death Syndrome: What Biological Anthropology Has Discovered About Normal Infant Sleep and Pediatric Sleep Medicine. *Yearbook of Physical Anthropology* 50:133-161.

lactation and birth spacing

Wood, J. Lactation and Birth Spacing. 1985. *Journal of Biosocial Science* 9, supplement:159-73.

nursing frequency and birth spacing

Konner, M. and Worthman, C. 1980. Nursing Frequency, Gonadal Function, and Birth Spacing Among !Kung Hunter-Gatherers. *Science* 207(4432):788-91.

composition of milk and frequency of suckling

Short, R. 1984. Breastfeeding. *Scientific American* 35.

nursing frequency and postpartum anovulation

Taylor, W. et al. 1991. Post-Partum Anovulation in Nursing Mothers. *Journal of Tropical Pediatrics* 37(6):286-292.

sympto-thermal method of NFP

Frank-Herrmann, P. et al. The effectiveness of a fertility awareness based method to avoid pregnancy in relation to a couple's sexual behaviour during the fertile time: a prospective longitudinal study. *Human Reproduction* 22(5):1310-1319.

Marquette method of NFP

Bouchard, T. et al. Efficacy of a new postpartum transition protocol for avoiding pregnancy. *J AM Board Fam Med* 26(1):35-44.

Recommended Online Resources

Spiritual

Holy Family Institute
www.vocations-holyfamily.com
www.hficoncord.com

Our Lady of La Leche Shrine
http://www.missionandshrine.org/la_leche.htm

Breastfeeding

Catholic Nursing Mothers League
www.catholicbreastfeeding.org
www.catholicbreastfeeding.blogspot.com

Ask Dr. Sears
www.askdrsears.com

LactMed
http://toxnet.nlm.nih.gov/cgi-bin/sis/htmlgen?LACT

Hale Publishing
http://www.ibreastfeeding.com/

Natural Family Planning

NFP International
www.nfpandmore.org

Marquette Method
nfp.marquette.edu

Creighton Model
www.creightonmodel.com

Billings Ovulation Method
www.thebillingsovulationmethod.com

USCCB Directory of NFP Providers
http://www.usccb.org/issues-and-action/marriage-and-family/natural-family-planning/awareness-week/nfp-providers.cfm

Parenting

Catholic Attachment Parenting
http://catholicap.com/

Intentional Catholic Parenting
http://intentionalcatholicparenting.com/

Recommended Books

Breastfeeding

Breastfeeding and Natural Child Spacing by Sheila Kippley

Breastfeeding and Catholic Motherhood by Sheila Kippley

The Seven Standards of Ecological Breastfeeding: The Frequency Factor by Sheila Kippley

The Baby Book, Revised Edition: Everything You Need to Know About Your Baby from Birth to Age Two (2013) by Dr. William Sears, Martha Sears, Dr. Robert Sears, and Dr. James Sears

"Breastfeeding and Bonding" chapter in *Mother and Infant* by Fr. William Virtue

Natural Family Planning

Natural Family Planning: The Complete Approach by John and Sheila Kippley

Parenting

Parenting with Grace by Gregory Popcak

The Discipline Book by Dr. William and Martha Sears

Nutrition

Fertility, Cycles and Nutrition by Marilyn Shannon

Eat Well, Lose Weight While Breastfeeding: The Complete Nutrition Book for Nursing Mothers by Eileen Behan

About the Author

Gina Peterson is a Catholic mother of four sons and one daughter, all whom she ecologically breastfed. She holds a BS in Mathematics and a BS in Basic Sciences from New Mexico Institute of Mining and Technology. She currently home educates her children and is a volunteer International Board Certified Lactation Consultant (IBCLC). She is also a perpetually professed member of the Holy Family Institute. Gina, her husband, and their children reside in Los Alamos, New Mexico.

www.ingramcontent.com/pod-product-compliance
Lightning Source LLC
Chambersburg PA
CBHW050356290526
45786CB00003B/1004